ADHD

A Proven Guide To Managing, Healing, And Coping With Adhd In Children And Teenagers

By

DR MARIA GUHIVER

TABLE OF CONTENTS

WHAT ARE ADHD

Attention-deficit hyperactivity problem (ADHD) is just one of the most common mental disorders affecting youngsters. ADHD additionally impacts lots of grownups. Signs of ADHD consist of negligence (not having the ability to keep emphasis), hyperactivity (an excess motion that is not fitting to the setup), and impulsivity (rash acts that occur in the minute without thought).

An approximated 8.4 percent of kids and also 2.5 percent of grownups have ADHD. ADHD is usually initially determined in school-aged kids when it brings about disruption in the class or troubles with schoolwork. It can, likewise, impact adults. It is extra usual among boys than women.

WHAT DOES IT MEAN TO HAVE ADHD?

Has anybody ever asked you if you have ADHD? Possibly you've also wondered on your own.

The only way to understand for sure is to see a physician. That's because the disorder has a variety of possible symptoms, and they can easily be puzzled with those of other conditions, like clinical depression or stress and anxiety.

Not sure whether you should obtain examined by a doc? If a number of these apply, you might require to get taken a look at it.

1. People state you're absent-minded.

Everyone loses cars and truck tricks or jackets from time to time. This kind of point happens commonly when you have ADHD. You may hang around looking for glasses, wallets, phones, as well as various other products each day. You may also forget to return call, area out on paying bills, or miss medical consultations.

2. People grumble that you do not pay attention to.

Most of us lose concentrate on a discussion from time to time, specifically, if there's a TV nearby or something else orders our interest. It takes place typically and also better with ADHD, also when there are no diversions around. Still, ADHD is even more than that.

3. You're typically behind schedule.

Time management is an ongoing challenge when you have ADHD It usually results in missed due dates or appointments unless you deal with preventing that.

4. You have difficulty concentrating.

Issues with interest, mainly focusing for extended periods or taking notice of details, is just one of the characteristics of the problem. Depression, anxiousness, and also addiction problems can likewise take a toll on your emphasis, as well as many individuals with ADHD have one or more of these problems, too. Your doctor can ask you inquiries to obtain to the base of what's causing your attention issues.

5. You leave points reversed.

Problems with interest and also memory can inconvenience to start or complete projects. Specifically, ones that you know will take a lot of focus to finish. This symptom can indicate depression, also.

6. You had behavior concerns as a child.

You need to have had attention as well as focus troubles as a kid to be identified with ADHD as an adult-- also if those early signs didn't feature an official diagnosis.

Individuals might have accused you of sluggard back in youth. Or they may have thought you had an additional problem like depression or stress and anxiety.

If you were detected with the disorder as a child, you might still have it. The signs change as you age, and also not everybody outgrows it.

7. You lack impulse control.

It is more than tossing a sweet bar right into your cart at the checkout line. It is doing something even though you understand it could have severe repercussions, like running a red light because you believe you can get away with it or otherwise being able to keep the peace when you have something to state, even though you recognize you should.

8. You can not get organized.

You might discover this more at work. You could have difficulty setting concerns, following up on tasks, and conference project deadlines.

9. You're fidgety.

Youngsters with ADHD are typically hyper, but adults are more likely to be fidgety or troubled. You might also chat too much, as well as to interrupt others.

10. You can't control your emotions.

You may be irritable or short-tempered, express frustration usually, feel indifferent or be susceptible to upset outbursts. ADHD can make it tough to handle awkward feelings or follow ideal habits when you're disturbed.

THE VARIOUS TYPES OF ADHD

Comprehending ADHD

Attention deficit disorder (ADHD) is a chronic condition. It primarily influences kids, yet can additionally impact adults. It can affect emotions, behaviors, and also the ability to learn brand-new things.

ADHD is separated right into three different types:

Neglectful type

Hyperactive-impulsive kind

Combination kind

Signs and symptoms will determine which sort of ADHD you have. To be identified with ADHD, symbols, and symptoms have to influence your day-to-day life.

Signs and symptoms can alter over time, so the kind of ADHD you have might change, as well. ADHD can be a long-lasting obstacle. Medicine and various other therapies can help improve your quality of life.

Three Types Of Symptoms

Each sort of ADHD is tied to several qualities. ADHD is identified by negligence and hyperactive-impulsive actions.

These Habits Frequently Present In The Adhering To Methods:

Negligence: obtaining sidetracked, having inadequate concentration and also organizational abilities

Impulsivity: disturbing, taking dangers

Hyperactivity: never appearing to slow down, talking as well as fidgeting, problems remaining on task

Everyone is different, so it's usual for two individuals to experience the very same signs in different ways. For example, these behaviors are typically mixed in young boys and also women. Children may be seen as more hyperactive, as well as girls may be silently unobserving.

Primarily apathetic ADHD

If you have this kind of ADHD, you may experience a lot more signs and symptoms of inattention than those of impulsivity as well as hyperactivity. You might battle with impulse control or attention deficit disorder at times. These aren't the primary attributes of neglectful ADHD.

People who experience apathetic actions commonly:

Miss details and also are sidetracked quickly

Get tired rapidly

Have difficulty concentrating on a solitary task

Have trouble organizing thoughts and also learning brand-new info

Lose pencils, papers, or various other things needed to finish a task

Don't appear to pay attention

Move gradually and also look as if they're daydreaming

Refine details much more slowly as well as much less appropriate than others

Have a problem following directions

Extra women are detected with neglectful kind ADHD than children.

Mainly Hyperactive-Impulsive ADHD

This kind of ADHD is defined by signs of impulsivity and attention deficit disorder. People with this type can present indications of inattention. However, it's not as significant as the various other symptoms.

People that are impulsive or hyper frequently:

Squirm, fidget, or feel restless

Have difficulty sitting still

Talk continuously

Touch as well as play with objects, even when inappropriate to the task handy

Have trouble engaging in quiet tasks

Are regularly "on the move."

Are impatient

Act out of turn and also don't think of repercussions of actions

Spout out solutions and too inappropriate remarks

Youngsters with hyperactive-impulsive kind ADHD can be an interruption in the classroom. They can make finding out more challenging on their own and even other students.

Mix ADHD

If you have the mix kind, it indicates that your signs and symptoms do not exclusively fall within the inattention or hyperactive-impulsive behavior. Instead, a mix of signs and symptoms from both of the categories is displayed.

Many people, with or without ADHD, experience some level of unobserving or spontaneous behavior. Yet it's extra dangerous in individuals with ADHD. The habits because place regularly as well as interferes with just how you function at home, institution, work, and also in social circumstances.

The Central Institute of Mental Health clarifies that many children have combination kind ADHD. The most usual symptom in preschool-age youngsters is attention deficit disorder.

CAUSES OF ADHD

The reason for ADHD in your kid can be traced back to the family members. The condition is genetically based, which in simple terms, implies your youngster may have acquired a few of your nerves genetics. Even though conditions in your home or college can add to it, they are not considered ADHD reasons.

There have been lots of scientific analyses that link physical attributes to the source of ADHD. These include gene makeup, absorbing toxic active ingredients, trauma to the mind, and responses to some artificial additive.

The make-up of your genetics:

Check out other members of your household. Did you recognize that even though three to five percent of kids are identified with ADHD, twenty-five percent of an ADHD child's relatives will certainly additionally have the condition? Scientific researches have also disclosed specific genes that have been linked to the root cause of ADHD!

Toxic components:

If you consumed alcohol or made use of tobacco products while you were expecting, and also you have an ADHD child, researches have indicated a possible link. A fetus will certainly absorb these poisonous compounds, which certainly can not be excellent. If your kid has been around constructing old frameworks, he may have been revealed to lead poisoning. Several of these toxic ingredients have been labeled as possible ADHD causes. When I was growing up on an arable farm, my Dad subjected me to DDT, which is currently outlawed in the USA. Possibly that added to my ADHD, and then my boy's.

Mind injury:

Most children, fortunately, don't come under this group; however, specific sorts of mental trauma can bring on ADHD signs. Scientific studies had shown that when an ADHD kid and a NON-ADHD kid had brain scans or an MRI, there were some distinctions in some regions of the mind. This would seem to show that the brain has something to do with the source of ADHD.

Food additives:

About 10 percent of ADHD kids show minimized signs when their sugar and additive intake has been reduced. Currently, right here is somewhat of a shock. While a lot of us, including me, tend to associate sugar with attention deficit disorder, there was no difference when children were given either sugar or a sugar replacement. That suggests that sugar doesn't contribute to ADHD signs.

Given that a lot of individuals have it in their heads that sugar triggers ADHD symptoms, they may see more signs after a youngster has some sugar. Studies reveal that moms and dads that believe that their children have been provided sugar (when they have been offered a substitute) are just as most likely to state that ADHD signs have worsened as parents of children that are given actual sugar.

Even if it is only regarded, a reduction in sugar consumption (or high fructose) can be beneficial.

A recent study has discovered that preservatives and also food coloring, which can be found in soft drinks as well as convenience food, significantly increase hyperactivity in children. So make sure you see what they are taking into their bodies.

Remember, ADHD triggers kids to act in unacceptable means. However, it doesn't need to be this approach. It is an extremely treatable problem. There are prescription drugs that work for the signs, natural remedies that attack the origin of the condition, nutritional control, and behavioral therapy. Do your study, and after that, do what is in your youngster's benefit.

ADHD SIGNS AND SYMPTOM

To assist you to recognize when your child may have attention deficit hyperactivity disorder, right here are some ADHD indicators you should understand.

1) Do you observe your child having difficulty in college jobs and other activities? The inability to concentrate as well as take note of instructions can result in reduced grades. Youngsters with ADHD also tend to stay clear of working on challenging tasks and try to make reasons whenever they need to do them.

2) Does it appear as if you're always searching for points that your kid has lost? Among the ADHD signs are forgetfulness and disorganization. Youngsters with ADHD typically shed things, fail to remember to do research, and leave their books at college.

3) Do you discover your kid always daydreaming? Those with ADHD commonly seem not to listen when they are talked with.

4) Is it tough for your kid to sit still? Fidgeting and also agonizing prevail ADHD indications amongst kids as they have a tough time remaining in their seats.

5) Does your child disrupt other children in his course due to his too much talking? Youngsters with ADHD

have a hard time keeping silent, even in situations where they are expected to do so.

6) Does your kid act as if an electric motor runs him? Continuously running, jumping, as well as climbing, are likewise ADHD indicators. Youngsters with ADHD have all this pent up power that requires to be released through activities like sporting activities.

7) Is your youngster fond of blurting out a solution to questions that are not yet also ended up? Spontaneity is one of the ADHD warning signs, and also, this can be possibly dangerous. For instance, they might do something like cross the street without looking.

8) Does your kid discover it hard waiting in line for his turn? Kids with ADHD often have this trouble, and they likewise interrupt other people who are speaking or in the middle of doing something.

These are ADHD indications that could prompt you to seek specialist help and assessment. Know that there are various therapy options available to you that are more secure and also even more expense efficient than prescription drugs.

The Four Warning Signs of ADHD Symptoms In Toddlers

Kids with ADHD do show signs and symptoms EARLY in their lives. Some parents are worried when their children seem to be a lot more spontaneous and also hyperactive compared with others at the very same age.

Here are a few of the signs and symptoms that youngsters with ADHD may display:

1. Rest disturbances: let's encounter it. Several 2 or 3 years of age are not good sleepers. Children with focus deficiency hyperactivity disorder are a lot more likely to have rest troubles than others, for example, waking up a lot more often throughout the night, and also having difficulty dropping asleep.

2. Severe hyper activeness: restless, running around non-stop till also tired to move, ruining things ... I bet these have taken place for most of our young children. However, kids with ADHD present these behaviors a lot more frequently and also exceptionally.

3. Inattention: Inattention is just one of the most ordinary signs and symptoms of ADHD. Youngsters with this problem are reported to be much more easily tired at games and playthings and are frequently distracted.

4. Hypersensitivity: correctly, how do you recognize if your kid is hypersensitive? Well, inspect the complying with signs. Do they refuse to put on the clothing of a specific material? Do they have aversions to foods of a particular texture? Some parents grumble that their kids just won't put on denim trousers because of the hard textiles. My very own child declined to eat bananas and eggs, considering that he was much less than one year of age.

If your young children have revealed the above indications for a minimum of 6 months, it is encouraged that you speak to their doctor regarding their condition.

When it comes to treatments for this neuro-behavioral problem, prescribed drugs might not appropriate for extremely young kids because of the possible harsh adverse effects.

GETTING AN ACCURATE DIAGNOSIS OF ADHD

Identifying ADHD: What you need to recognize

Are you quickly sidetracked, hopelessly chaotic, or regularly absent-minded and questioning if attention deficit disorder (ADHD) is responsible? Do you take a look at your rambunctious, restless child, and also believe it might be ADHD? Before you leap to verdicts, remember that identifying ADHD isn't somewhat that simple. By themselves, none of the signs and symptoms of focus deficiency disorder are irregular. Most individuals feel scattered, unfocused, or agitated, sometimes. Also, chronic attention deficit disorder or distractibility doesn't always equivalent to ADHD.

There is no solitary clinical, physical, or another test for identifying ADHD, previously called ADD. To determine if you or your youngster has ADHD, a doctor or other health and wellness professionals will certainly need to be entailed, as well as you can expect them to make use of a variety of different tools: a list of signs and symptoms, response to questions concerning past and existing troubles, or a medical examination to eliminate other causes for signs and symptoms.

Keep in mind that the signs of ADHD, such as focus issues as well as hyperactivity, can be puzzled with various other disorders as well as medical problems, consisting of discovering handicaps as well as emotional issues, which require different treatments. Just because it looks like ADHD does not indicate it is, so obtaining a comprehensive analysis and medical diagnosis is essential.

Making the ADHD medical diagnosis

ADHD looks different in everyone, so there is a wide variety of criteria to help health and wellness experts reach a medical diagnosis. It is essential to be open as well as sincere with the expert performing your analysis to ensure that he or she can get to one of the most precise conclusions.

To obtain an ADHD medical diagnosis, you or your child should display a combination of intense ADHD characteristic symptoms, namely attention deficit disorder, impulsivity, or negligence. The mental health specialist analyzing the trouble will certainly additionally check out the following variables:

How extreme are the symptoms? To be identified with ADHD, the symptoms have to harm you or your kid's life. Generally, people who really have ADHD have significant issues in one or more locations of their life, such as their career, funds, or household responsibilities.

When did the symptoms begin? Given that ADHD starts in childhood years, the physician or specialist will consider precisely how very early the symptoms appeared. If you are an adult, can you trace the signs back to your childhood?

The length of time have the symptoms been troubling you or your child? Signs need to have been going on for a minimum of 6 months before ADHD can be detected.

When and also where do the signs and symptoms appear? The signs of ADHD must exist in numerous setups, such as in the house and even college. If the signs only show up in one atmosphere, it is not likely that ADHD is at fault.

Usual signs and symptoms of ADHD

Signs of negligence

Often fails to give close attention to information or makes mistakes

Commonly has problem maintaining focus while completing jobs or partaking in tasks

Often does not seem to listen when spoken with straight

Usually does not follow through with instructions as well as fails to finish schoolwork or work environment obligations

Commonly has trouble organizing tasks and also activities

Usually avoids, disapproval or is reluctant to take part in jobs that require continual psychological effort

Loses products necessary of employment or activities

Is easily distracted by nonessential stimulations

Is usually absent-minded in daily tasks

Signs and symptoms of hyperactivity and also impulsivity

Typically fidgets with or taps hands and feet, or squirms in seat

Commonly leaves the position in scenarios when staying seated is anticipated

Frequently unable to play or engage in leisure activities quietly

Often runs and also climbs up in situations where it is improper (in adolescents or adults, might be limited to feeling uneasy).

Is often "on the go," acting as if "driven by an electric motor."

Commonly blurts out responses before concern has been completed.

Typically has difficulty waiting their turn.

Frequently interrupts or invades others.

Typically talks excessively.

discovering an expert who can identify ADHD.

Certified professionals trained in detecting ADHD can consist of medical psychologists, medical professionals, or scientific, social employees. Choosing an expert can appear puzzling. The adhering to actions can aid you to locate the appropriate person to assess you or your child.

Obtain suggestions.

Specialists and good friends you depend on may refer you to a specific specialist. Ask questions concerning their choice as well as check out their suggestions.

Do your homework.

Figure out the specialist qualification as well as the academic degrees of the professionals you are exploring. Preferably, talk with former people as well as customers, and also learn what their experience was.

Feel secure.

Feeling comfortable with the expert is an integral part of selecting the best person to review you. Attempt to be yourself, ask concerns, and also be honest with the specialist. You might require to speak with a couple of professionals before finding the person that is finest for you.

Check rate as well as an insurance policy.

Discover how much the professional will undoubtedly charge as well as if your medical insurance will cover part or every one of the ADHD analysis. Some insurance plan cover assessment for ADHD from one type of specialist, yet not from one more.

Detecting ADHD in grownups.

Many people only discover that they have ADHD actually when they become adults. Some learn after their youngsters obtain a medical diagnosis. As they end up being enlightened regarding the problem, they likewise understand that they have it. For others, the signs lastly surpass their coping skills, triggering substantial adequate issues in their daily life that they look for aid. If you recognize the symptoms and signs of ADHD in on your own, set up a visit with a psychological wellness professional for an analysis. Once you make that first visit, feeling somewhat anxious regarding it is normal.

If you recognize what to anticipate, the process for reviewing ADHD isn't complicated or scary. Several professionals will begin by asking you to fill in and return questionnaires before an assessment. You'll probably be asked to call a person near to you that will certainly additionally participate in several of the evaluation. To establish if you have ADHD, you can anticipate the specialist conducting the assessment to do any type of or all of the following:

Ask you about your symptoms, consisting of how long they've been troubling you as well as any troubles they've triggered in the past.

Administer ADHD examinations, such as symptom lists and also attention-span examinations.

Speak with a relative or somebody close to you about your symptoms.

Offer you a medical exam to eliminate other physical causes for the signs.

Should I be tested for grown-up ADHD?

If you have substantial problems with any of the following categories, you might want to get assessed for ADHD.

Work or occupation: shedding or stopping work frequently.

Job or school: not performing up to your ability or capacity.

Daily jobs: inability to do family duties, pay bills promptly, organize points.

Relationships: failing to remember important things, having difficulty completing jobs, obtaining upset over small issues.

Emotions: experiencing recurring stress as well as fear because you don't satisfy objectives or meet responsibilities.

It is detecting ADHD in kids.

When looking for a diagnosis for your child, having a "team attitude" might aid. You are not alone, as well as with the help of others. You can obtain to the bottom of your child's battles. Together with specialists trained in diagnosing ADHD, you can aid produce a swift and also exact analysis that results in treatment.

Your role as a parent.

When looking for a diagnosis for your kid, you are your kid's ideal supporter, as well as the most crucial source of support. As moms and dads in this procedure, your roles are both emotional as well as useful.

You can need psychological assistance for your child throughout the analysis procedure.

Guarantee that your kid sees the best professional and also get a second opinion if required.

Provide unique and handy information for doctors/specialists, including open and also honest answers to questions about your child's history and existing adjustment.

Display the speed and accuracy of the analysis.

The Physician's Or Expert's Function.

Usually, more than one specialist examines a kid for ADHD signs. Physicians, medical and also institution psychologists, scientific,, social workers, speech-language pathologists, learning professionals, as well as teachers,, might each play an essential role in the ADHD assessment.

Similar to grownups, there are no lab or imaging examinations available to make a medical diagnosis; instead, medical professionals base their verdicts on the evident signs and symptoms and also by dismissing other disorders. The expert that conducts your child's analysis will ask you a range of questions that you should address honestly and too freely. They may additionally.

Acquire a detailed clinical and also family history.

Order or perform a necessary physical and neurological exam.

Lead a thorough interview with you, your youngster, and your kid's teacher(s).

Usage standardized testing tools for ADHD.

Observe your child at play or college.

necessary

Obtaining your child reviewed for ADHD

Doctors, specialists, ADHD examinations-- it might all feel a little frustrating to go after diagnosis for your youngster. You can take a lot of the turmoil out of the procedure with the following practical actions.

Make an appointment with a professional.

Aa parent, you can initiate testing for ADHD in support of your child. The earlier you arrange this consultation, the earlier you can get assist for their ADHD.

Speak to your kid's college.

Call your child's principal as well as speak straight as well as freely regarding your pursuit of a medical diagnosis Public colleges are needed by regulation to assist you, as well as in many cases, the staff wants to aid enhance your child's life at college.

Give professionals the full photo.

When you are asked the complicated concerns regarding your child's actions, be sure to address truthfully. Your viewpoint fundamental to the assessment procedure.

Keep points relocating?

You are your kid's supporter, as well as have the power to stop hold-ups in obtaining a medical diagnosis. Check-in with physicians or professionals adequately frequently to see where you are in the process.

If required, get a second opinion. If there is any type of uncertainty that your child has obtained a comprehensive or proper analysis, you can look for one more professional's help.

Recognizing an ADHD diagnosis.

It's regular to feel upset or frightened by a diagnosis of ADHD. Yet keep in mind that getting a diagnosis can be the initial step towards making life better. As soon as you recognize what you're managing, you can begin getting treatment-- which indicates taking control of signs and symptoms as well as feeling even more confident in every area of life.

An ADHD medical diagnosis might feel like a label. However, it might be extra valuable to consider it as an explanation. The diagnosis explains why you might have fought with life abilities such as paying attention, following directions, listening very carefully, organization-- things that seem ahead conveniently to other individuals.

In this feeling, getting a medical diagnosis can be an alleviation. You can relax much more comfortable recognizing that it wasn't idleness or a lack of knowledge standing in your or your child's means, however rather a disorder that you can find out just how to handle.

Additionally, remember that an ADHD diagnosis is not a sentence for a lifetime of suffering. Some people have only mild signs and symptoms, while others experience even more pervasive issues. despite where you or your child land on this range, there are many steps you can take to manage your signs and symptoms.

Co-existing problems and ADHD.

It is essential to recognize that an ADHD diagnosis does not dismiss other psychological health conditions. The following terms are not component of an ADHD diagnosis but sometimes co-occur with ADHD, or get confused with it:

Anxiousness-- Excessive fear that happens frequently and also is challenging to manage. Symptoms include feeling restless or on the side, quickly tired out, anxiety attack, irritability, muscle mass tension, and sleeping disorders.

Clinical depression-- symptoms consist of sensations of pessimism, helplessness, and also self-loathing, in addition to changes in rest and too eating behaviors and even a loss of passion in activities you used to appreciate.

Learning impairment-- Problems with analysis, composing, or math. When provided standardized tests, the trainee's capability or intelligence is considerably higher than their achievement.

Chemical abuse-- The impulsivity and also behavioral issues that commonly accompany ADHD can lead to alcohol and even medication issues.

Getting help after an ADHD diagnosis

A medical diagnosis of ADHD can be an excellent wake-up telephone call-- it can provide you the added push you need to look for aid for the signs and symptoms that are hindering your joy and success. If you or your child is detected with ADHD, don't wait to begin therapy. The earlier you start dealing with the symptoms, the better.

Taking care of ADHD takes a job.

Discovering the right therapies for you or your kid is a process-- one that takes some time, perseverance, and also experimentation. But you can aid on your own along the road by keeping the adhering to goals in mind: discovering as much as you can around ADHD, obtaining a lot of support, and also adopting healthy and balanced lifestyle behaviors.

ADHD Is Treatable.

Don't surrender hope. With the right treatment and assistance, you or your kid will certainly have the ability to get the signs of ADHD under control as well as develop the life that you desire.

Therapy is your very own responsibility.

It's up to you to do something about it to take care of the signs and symptoms of ADHD. Wellness specialists can help, but inevitably, the obligation lies in your very own hands.

Learning all you can around ADHD is vital.

Understanding the condition will assist you in making informed choices regarding all aspects of your or your youngster's life and also treatment.

Support makes all the difference.

While therapy depends on you, sustain from others can aid you to remain inspired as well as get you with bumpy rides.

GETTING GOING WITH YOUR ACTION PLAN

Organize the cooking area. Clean out the garage. Reach the fitness center. Send out thank you cards. Meal prep for the week. Foot the bill. ADHDers usually have lots they 'd like to obtain done, yet somehow their to-do lists never receive any kind of much shorter. Why? Since merely deciding to do something isn't enough. You require an action strategy that consists of the What, How, Where, When, Who, as well as Why for each task on your listing.

Preparation isn't something that comes naturally for many individuals with ADHD. That's because ADHDers commonly have weak exec feature abilities which regulate the capability to plan, arrange, and also handle your time successfully. Consequently, day-to-day jobs may go by the wayside, or you might find on your own unprepared for those tasks you do begin as well as inevitably don't complete. Fortunately is with some preparation ahead of time, you'll be far better able to successfully tackle those to-do list items that never appear to obtain done.

Step 1: The What

When you prepare for any job, start with the end in mind: What EXACTLY are you attempting to achieve? What's your endgame? Exactly how will you know you've completed the job at hand? You require to recognize where you're going before you can plan on how you'll arrive.

Step 2: The How

How will I obtain this job done? Think about this action as your pre-plan. To put it, what factors require to be consisted of in your plan? Do you require materials? Do you need to work with the task at a specific time or in a particular area? Will you require help and additional details to get going? Are there multiple steps included? Accurately how will you manage interruptions and also various other possible obstructions?

Step 3: The Where

Where will you work with your job? This might seem like a no-brainer depending upon the activity; however, the area can be a crucial element when you have ADHD. You might need total silence with no disturbances to obtain points done or you might discover that you function well with a little bit of an ambient "buzz" around you and also are most productive functioning in your neighborhood coffee store. Even if you prepare to operate at home, you'll intend to consider area: The cooking area table? Your work desk? On the couch in front of the TV?

Step 4: The When

Many individuals with ADHD deal with time monitoring, consisting of time ignorance, which implies you might have trouble accurately evaluating how much time something will take to complete. You may have additionally uncovered that if you do not set up or take a moment to do something, it doesn't get done. That's why "the When" is a necessary action in your planning. When do you prepare to service your task? When does it require to be completed? If there are numerous actions, what are the due dates for those? Be as precise as possible and set a pointer in either your planner or your phone, or you're sure to forget or else.

Tip 5: The Who

You'll want to think of what else requires to be a part of your plan. Take into consideration whether you'll need someone else's support with all or component of your task. If you do, it'll be essential to collaborate with them so they'll be offered. You may likewise want to think about whether or not the job, at the very least in part, could be dealt with by another person, either in your family or an outside specialist.

Step 6: The Why

Last, however, absolutely not least, consider "the Why." When your inspiration to start or complete a product on your to-do list begins to wane., you'll intend to remember your "why." Why is completing this job vital to you? What do you want to get because of this? How will your life be more straightforward? How will you feel when it's done? Remembering your "why" will assist you in pressing via those "I don't feel like it" moments.

As the stating goes, "A goal without a strategy is just a desire." It takes more than merely deciding to do something to, in fact, obtain it done. Taking the, use your time more effectively, as well as stay on track.

COPING WITH COMMON PROBLEMS IF YOU ARE A PARENT OF A CHILD WITH ADHD

Learn what you can do to supervise your kid's habits and bargain with common ADHD challenges.

How to aid your youngster with ADHD

Life with a kid or teenager with attention deficit hyperactivity disorder (ADHD or ADD) can be aggravating, even overwhelming. As a parent you can aid your youngster got rid of day-to-day challenges, direct their energy into favorable sectors, and also bring better tranquility to your household As well as the earlier and a lot more consistently you address your child's troubles, the higher chance they have for success in life.

Children with ADHD usually have deficiencies in decision-making features: the ability to think and prepare in advance, organize, control impulses, and also full tasks. That means you require to take over as the executive, providing added assistance while your child progressively acquires executive abilities of their own.

Although the signs and symptoms of ADHD can be absolutely nothing short of annoying, it's crucial to remember that the kid who is neglecting, irritating, or awkward, you are not acting willfully. Youngsters with

ADHD wish to sit silently; they intend to make their areas neat and also organized; they intend to do every little thing their parent says to do-- but they don't know exactly how to make these points occur.

If you keep in mind that having ADHD is equally as discouraging for your child, it will be a great deal simpler to respond in favorable, supportive ways. With perseverance, empathy, and also lots of assistance, you can manage childhood years ADHD while taking pleasure in a steady, pleasing home.

ADHD and your family members.

Before you can help effectively moms and dad a child with ADHD, it's vital to recognize the impact of your youngster's signs on the family members in its entirety. Children with ADHD exhibit a multitude of habits that can interfere with domesticity. They often do not "listen to" adult directions, so they do not obey them. They're disordered and also easily distracted, keeping another member of the family waiting. Or they start tasks as well as fail to remember to complete them-- not to mention clean up after them. Kids with impulsivity problems typically interrupt conversations, demand interest at inappropriate times, and talk before they assume, claiming thoughtless or embarrassing points. It's usually hard to get them to bed and also to rest. Hyperactive kids may tear around your home and even put themselves in physical danger.

Due to these habits, brothers or sisters of youngsters with ADHD deal with a variety of difficulties. Their needs commonly get much less interest than those of youngsters with ADHD. They may be ticked off much more sharply when they err, as well as their successes may be less renowned or considered provided. They may be enlisted as assistant parents-- and condemned if the sibling with ADHD misbehaves under their supervision. Consequently, brothers or sisters may locate their love for a sibling or sister with ADHD mixed with envy and also resentment.

The need to monitor a youngster with ADHD can be physically and mentally exhausting. Your child's failure to "listen" can lead to aggravation and that aggravation to rage-- adhered to by a sense of guilt concerning being angry at your kid. Your youngster's behavior can make you nervous and worried. If there's a fundamental difference between your personality which of your child with ADHD, their behavior can be particularly challenging to accept.

To satisfy the challenges of elevating a youngster with ADHD, you should be able to master a mix of concern and uniformity. Staying in a house that gives both loves as well as the structure is the very best point for a child or teenager who is discovering to manage ADHD.

ADHD parenting suggestion 1: Stay favorable as well as healthy on your own

As a mom and dad, you set the phase for your child's psychological and physical health and wellness. You have control over most of the factors that can positively influence the signs of your kid's problem.

Keep a favorable attitude. Your most beautiful properties for assisting your child in satisfying the challenges of ADHD are your favorable mindset as well as sound judgment. When you are calm and concentrated, you are much more likely to be able to connect with your kid, assisting him or her to be tranquil as well as focused.

Keep points in perspective. Keep in mind that your child's behavior is related to a disorder. A lot of the time, it is not intentional. Hold on to your sense of humor. What's awkward today might be a fun family member's tale ten years from now.

Don't sweat the tiny things as well as want to make some concessions. One task left undone isn't a massive deal when your child has finished two others plus the day's research. If you are a nit-picker, you will not just be dissatisfied continuously but also create impossible assumptions for your child with ADHD.

Rely on your youngster. Think of or make a written checklist of whatever that declares, significant, as well as distinct regarding your kid. Depend on that; your child can find out, alter, fully grown, and be successful. Declare this trust fund every day as you clean your teeth or make your coffee.

Self-care

Woman relaxing by home window As your kid's good example and also an essential resource of toughness, it is crucial that you live a healthy life. If you are overtired or have lacked patience, you run the risk of losing sight of the framework and assistance you have so carefully set up for your child with ADHD.

Seek assistance.

Among one of the most vital things to keep in mind in rearing a child with ADHD is that you do not have to do it alone. Speak with your child's physicians, specialists, and instructors. Join an orderly support system for moms and dads of kids with ADHD. These groups supply an online forum for providing as well as obtaining advice and give a safe place to air vent feelings as well as share experiences.

Take breaks.

Buddies and family members can be fantastic concerning using to babysit, but you may feel guilty about leaving your youngster or leaving the volunteer with a youngster with ADHD. Next time, approve their offer and also talk about honestly just how ideal for managing your kid.

Take care of yourself.

Consume right, workout, and discover ways to decrease stress and anxiety, whether it suggests taking a nighttime bath or practicing early morning meditation. If you do get ill, recognize it as well as get assistance.

Suggestion 2: Establish structure and also adhere to it

Kids with ADHD are most likely to succeed in finishing tasks when the tasks happen in foreseeable patterns and foreseeable places. Your work is to produce and suffer structure in your house to ensure that your kid understands what to anticipate as well as what they are expected to do.

Tips for assisting your kid with ADHD keep focused and also arranged:

Follow a regimen.

It is essential to establish a time and an area for every little thing to assist the child with ADHD comprehend as well as meet assumptions. Develop basic and also predictable routines for dishes, homework, play, as well as a bed. Have your youngster set out garments for the following early morning before going to bed, and also make sure whatever she or he needs to take to school is in a unique place, prepared to get hold of.

Usage clocks and timers.

Consider placing clocks all through the house, with a large one in your youngster's room. Permit enough time for what your child requires to do, such as research or getting ready in the early morning. Make use of a timer for homework or transitional times, such as in between finishing up play as well as preparing for bed.

Streamline your child's schedule. It is excellent to stay clear of quiet time, but a child with ADHD may end up being much more distracted and "end up" if there are lots of after-school tasks. You might require to make adjustments to the kid's after-school commitments based on the private kid's capacities and also the needs of particular activities.

Create a peaceful area.

Make confident your youngster has a quiet, private room of their very own. A deck or a bedroom job well, as long as it's not the same place as the youngster goes for a break.

Do your ideal to be neat and also arranged. Set up your residence in an orderly way. Make sure your youngster understands that every little thing has its place. Lead by instance with neatness and company as much as feasible.

Stay clear of troubles by keeping children with ADHD hectic!

For children with ADHD, still, time might intensify their signs and also create chaos in your house. It is essential to maintain a kid with ADHD busy without overdoing a lot of points that the kid ends up being overwhelmed.

Authorize your child up for a sport, art class, or music. In your home, arrange straightforward tasks that fill your youngster's time. These can be tasks like aiding you to prepare, playing a board game with a sibling, or illustrating. Try not to over-rely on the television or computer/video games as time-fillers. However, TV and also video games are increasingly violent and also may only enhance your kid's signs of ADHD.

Tip 3: Encourage movement as well as rest

Family playing basketball Children with ADHD commonly have the power to shed. Organized sports and various other exercises can assist them in obtaining their energy out in healthy and balanced means and concentrate their interest in specific activities as well as abilities. The advantages of training are unlimited: it boosts focus, reduces depression as well as anxiousness, and promotes mental development. Most importantly for children with focus deficiencies, however, is the reality that exercise leads to far better sleep, which in turn can also lower the signs and symptoms of ADHD.

Find a sporting activity that your child will enjoy, and that fits their stamina. For example, sporting activities such as softball that involve a lot of "downtime" are not the very best suitable for kids with focus troubles. Individual or group sporting activities like basketball and hockey that call for constant movement are better options. Youngsters with ADHD might likewise take advantage of training in martial arts (such as tae kwon do) or yoga exercise, which boosts mental control as they work out the body.

Not enough rest can make any person less conscientious, yet it can be extremely destructive for kids with ADHD. Youngsters with ADHD need at least as much rest as their untouched peers but often tend not to get what they need. Their interest problems can result in overstimulation as well as problems sleeping. A constant, very early bedtime is one of the most practical strategies to battle this issue. However, it might not fix it.

Assist your child to improve remainder by checking out one or more of the adhering to strategies:

Decline tv time and also enhance your youngster's activities and exercise degrees during the day.

Eliminate Caffeine From Your Child's Diet.

Produce a buffer time to decrease down the task degree for an hour or two before bedtime. Locate quieter activities such as coloring, reviewing, or playing quietly.

Spend ten mins cuddling with your child. It will build a sense of love as well as protection as well as give time to cool down.

Usage Lavender Or Other Aromas In Your Child's Room. The scent may aid in relaxing your youngster.

Usage leisure tapes as history sound for your youngster when falling asleep. There are several ranges available consisting of nature audios and calming songs. Youngsters with ADHD commonly locate "white noise" to be relaxing. You can develop white sound by placing a radio on fixed or running an electric follower. 2 youngsters running outside

The advantages of "green time" in kids with focus deficit condition

Research shows that kids with ADHD gain from hanging out in nature. Children experience a better decrease in signs and symptoms of ADHD when they play in a park loaded with the yard and also trees than on a concrete play area. Bear in mind of this promising as well as a primary method for managing ADHD. Even in cities, many family members have access to parks as well as various other all-natural setups. Join your youngsters in this "eco-friendly time"-- you'll additionally obtain a much-deserved breath of fresh air for yourself.

Pointer 4: Set Clear Expectations And Rules

Children with ADHD need consistent policies that they can understand as well as comply with. Make the rules of actions for the family straightforward and clear. Jot down the guidelines and hang them up in an area where your kid can easily read them.

Children with ADHD react particularly well to arranged systems of incentives as well as effects. It's essential to describe what will occur when the regulations are complied with as well as when they are damaged. Stick to your system: comply with through each as well as every time with an incentive or a consequence.

As you develop these permanent structures, remember that kids with ADHD usually obtain objection. Watch permanently actions-- as well as praise it. Praise is especially crucial for kids that have ADHD because they typically get so little of it. These kids receive an adjustment, remediation, and grievances concerning their behavior-- but little favorable reinforcement.

A smile, favorable comment, or various other benefits from you can improve the attention, focus as well as impulse control of your youngster with ADHD. Do your ideal to focus on giving positive praise for proper behavior as well as job conclusion, while providing as few adverse responses as feasible to unsuitable habits or inadequate job efficiency. Compensate your youngster for small success that you could take for granted in one more kid.

Making Use Of Rewards as well as Consequences

Incentives

Reward your youngster with benefits, appreciation, or activities, rather than with food or toys.

Change awards frequently. Children with ADHD obtain bored if the benefit is always the same.

Make a chart with points or celebrities awarded for the right actions, so your youngster has a beautiful reminder of their successes.

Immediate rewards function far better than the pledge of a future reward, however small benefits causing a huge one can likewise function.

Always follow through with an incentive.

Repercussions

Effects must be defined in advance and take place right away after your kid has misbehaved.

Try breaks as well as the elimination of benefits as repercussions for misbehavior.

Remove your kid from situations as well as environments that activate unacceptable habits.

When your youngster is mischievous, ask what she or he could have done instead. After that, have your child show it.

Always follow through with an effect.

Pointer 5: Help your kid consume right

Diet regimen is not a straight root cause of attention shortage condition, yet food can and does influence your kid's psychological state, which in turn seems to affect actions. Monitoring and also changing what, when, and also how much your youngster eats can help reduce the signs of ADHD.

All youngsters take advantage of fresh foods, routine mealtimes, and also staying away from fast food. These tenets are especially real for kids with ADHD, whose spontaneity and distractedness can result in missed out on dishes, disordered eating, as well as over-eating.

Children with ADHD are infamous for not eating regularly. Without parental guidance, these youngsters could not eat for hours and afterward binge on whatever is about. The result of this pattern can be ruining the kid's physical and also psychological wellness.

Prevent harmful consuming practices by scheduling regular nourishing meals or snacks for your kid no more than three hours apart. Physically, a youngster with ADHD needs a habitual intake of healthy and balanced food; emotionally, mealtimes are a required break and a setup rhythm to the day.

Do away with the junk foods in your home.

Place fatty and also sweet foods off-limits when eating in restaurants.

Switch off tv shows riddled with junk-food ads.

Give your child an everyday vitamin-and-mineral supplement.

Idea 6: Teach your kid just how to make friends

Kids with ADHD typically have a problem with necessary social communications. They might battle with reading social cues, talk way too much, disturb regularly, or come off as hostile or "also extreme." Their family member's psychological immaturity can make them stand apart among children their very own age, as well as make them targets for hostile teasing.

Do not forget, though, that lots of children with ADHD are incredibly smart as well as imaginative as well as will at some point figure out for themselves how to get along with others as well as place people who aren't suitable as good friends. Character traits that could annoy parents and also educators may come throughout to peers as amusing and too lovely.

Helping a youngster with ADHD boost social abilities

It's tough for children with ADHD to discover social skills as well as social rules. You can aid your youngster with ADHD, become a far better listener, learn to review individuals' faces as well as body language, and also engage even more efficiently in teams.

Speak delicately, however, honestly with your child concerning their difficulties as well as just how to make modifications.

Role-play different social scenarios with your child. Trade frequently functions as well as attempts to make it enjoyable.

Beware to select buddies for your child with comparable language as well as physical skills.

Welcome only one or two friends at once in the beginning. See them carefully while they play and also have a zero-tolerance policy for hitting, pushing as well as screaming.

Make time as well as an area for your youngster to play, and also compensate for significant play behaviors commonly.

DISCIPLINE, COMMUNICATION AND THE ADHD CHILD

Parenting Dos and Don'ts: ADHD and Discipline

Do: Shift Your Mindset

With ADHD, typical methods of the technique aren't always the most effective fit. Shift your attitude from "I need to self-control my child" and also get interested in how to aid them to boost their skills. Taking a mindset of, "What can I do to aid them" instead of "How can I obtain them to do what I desire" is a game-changer.

Do: Ask Yourself This Question

Are your child's habits mischievous? Put, is he purposefully making a poor selection, or dealing with the impulsivity that usually comes with ADHD? A lot of children that have ADHD understand what they must do but can not get themselves to do it. If you select to see it as something they wish to do, however, is having a hard time with, you're more likely to lead favorably rather than punish.

Do not: Yell

If your little girl obtained sidetracked and also really did not do her homework, take a deep breath. If you yell, it will not alter anything. She'll close down and also not listen to anything you state. Even if it does seem to "work" in the short-term, it's harmful because your child is just motivated by worry. You desire your child to trust you. Don't design what it looks like to lose control.

Do: Be Brief

When you communicate with a youngster that has ADHD, obtain his attention. Keep it brief and also comfortable. If you make a demand, ensure he recognizes it. If it's a high demand-- It's time to speak about your grades, for instance-- surprise the conversation over a collection of days or weeks. It gives him time to process in amongst.

Do not: Think Too Far Ahead

Even if your kid does not finish tidying up his unpleasant space today doesn't indicate he'll never see points via. You do not need to show your youngster to master every little thing today. With your support as well as assistance, he'll find out each ability when he's ready. Construct your method to the future rather than worrying about what it could look like.

Do: Learn and also Be Compassionate

You can not see the internal functions of your kid's brain. All you see is your youngster's habits. That can be frustrating as well as complicated. Much like in any other attempting situation, it assists in being educated and understanding. Check out all you can around ADHD from relied on resources, so you recognize the problem, and also be compassionate with your kid as well as on your own.

Don't: Ask Too Much of Your Child

Children with ADHD can not regulate themselves in addition to various other children the very same age. They may do something well one day and also not do it well the next. It's way too much to ask a kid with ADHD to be consistent. You'll both feel a lot better if you fulfill your kid where she or he remains in any provided minute.

Do: Celebrate the Wins

Take notice of what goes well. Maybe your child increased his qualities, also if he still leaves all the lights on in your home. Change your perspective so that you see as well as commemorate what worked out. Reinforce the good as opposed to just house on what you 'd like to be various. When your child does what they understand well, highlight the initiative, and also what caused the actions. "You obtained your homework done. You need to feel so pleased with on your own. How did that take place so we can keep this going?"

Do not: Address Every Little Thing

Kids with ADHD are wrong often. They get redirected throughout the day, daily. If you take on everything regularly, it'll use you both out. Select one or two habits to deal with and let the remainder opt for now. You'll reach them at some point. This way, your youngster won't have that "I can't do anything best" feeling regularly.

Do: Coach and also Collaborate

You wouldn't anticipate your youngster to comprehend precisely how to play football without an instructor. You likewise can not expect them to manage themselves when their brains aren't wired to inform them exactly how. Train as well as collaborate with your child so that they can practice abilities as well as decision-making in a risk-free environment. Exercise with expressions like, "How do you assume we should manage this scenario?" Listen and afterward determine what's most beautiful.

Do: Look for the Opportunities

Your child can not sit still at supper. She maintains popping up and running about. However, she's been handling her behavior at school throughout the day and also is tired. Change your expectations, so she does not feel pity for making mistakes. Set an objective for her to settle down for merely 2 mins. Or select it as well as let her be the person that obtains the added catsup and removes plates as everyone surfaces.

Do: Punish Every Child Fairly

If you have more than one child as well as they do not all have ADHD, their effects might need to be various.

That can be a complicated region for moms and dads. Tell all your kids that you're a team, and also consequences will undoubtedly be reasonable; however, not regularly the same. Show concern when any one of your youngsters feels upset. Say, "I recognize this might be hard for you to accept." Do: Take Care of Yourself

ADHD actions can be tough to deal with. When you're tranquil as well as rested, you can deal with more and also handle it better. It may suggest you cut down on dedications and readjust your timetable and standards. Self-care-- like exercise, rest, and a great diet regimen- - is additionally vital. This way, you're better organized to help your household-- as well as on your own-- flourish.

HANDLING HOMEWORK FOR A CHILD WITH ADHD

Establishing your kid for college success

The classroom setting can present obstacles for a kid with attention deficit disorder (ADHD or ADD). The actual tasks these trainees find the hardest-- resting still, paying attention quietly, focusing-- are the ones they are called for to do all day long. Maybe most frustrating of all is that most of these children want to have the ability to find out and behave like their untouched peers. Neurological deficits, not hesitation, maintain children with attention deficit disorder from finding out in conventional means.

As a parent, you can aid your child deal with these deficits and also conquer the difficulties college develops. You can work with your child to put into action practical approaches for discovering both in and out of the classroom as well as connect with teachers about just how your youngster learns ideal. With regular support, the following strategies can aid your child delight in finding out, satisfy instructional difficulties-- and experience success at college and also past.

Tips for working with educators

Remember that your child's educator has a full plate: along with taking care of a group of kids with unique individualities as well as learning styles, they can likewise expect to have at the very least one student with ADHD. Teachers might attempt their best to assist your kid with a focus deficiency disorder find out accurately. However, parental participation can substantially boost your youngster's education. You have the power to maximize your kid's possibilities for success by supporting the actions absorbed in the class. If you can work with and also help your kid's educator, you can directly affect the knowledge of your child with ADHD at school.

There are several methods you can collaborate with instructors to keep your youngster on a course at school. With each other, you can assist your child with ADHD learn to find their feet in the classroom and also work successfully through the challenges of the school day. As a parent, you are your child's supporter. For your kid to do well in the classroom, you must connect their demands to the adults at school. It is equally vital for you to listen to what the educators and also various other college officials have to state.

You can ensure that interaction with your youngster's college is useful as well as practical. Try to keep in mind that your joint function is figuring out how to ideal assist your youngster be successful in school. Whether you talk over the phone, email, or fulfill personally, make an initiative to be calm, details, and, most importantly, positive-- a unique perspective can go a lengthy method when communicating with the institution.

Plan in advance.

You can prepare to consult with school officials or instructors before the school year even starts. If the year has begun, strategy to talk with a teacher or therapist on at least a month-to-month basis.

Make meetings occur. Settle on a time that benefits both you as well as your kid's teacher and adhere to it. If it's hassle-free, satisfy in your kid's classroom so you can obtain a feeling of your kid's physical learning setting.

Produce goals with each other.

Discuss your hopes for your kid's institution's success. With each other, make a note of individual as well as practical objectives as well as speak about exactly how to help your youngster reach them.

Listen thoroughly.

Like you, your child's teacher wants to see your child be successful at school. Listen to what they have to say-- even if it is sometimes difficult to listen to. Understanding your youngster's obstacles in college is crucial to discovering remedies that work.

Share information.

You recognize your child's history, as well as your kid's instructor, sees them daily: with each other, you have a lot of details that can result in a far better understanding of your child's difficulties. Share your observations easily, as well as motivate your youngster's instructors to do the same.

Ask the hard questions and offer a complete picture.

Make sure to detail any medicines your youngster takes and describe any other therapies. Share with your kid's instructor which methods work well-- and also which do not-- for your youngster in the house. Ask if your kid is having any troubles in the institution, including on the playground. Learn if your child is qualified for any special services to help with knowing.

Creating as well as using a behavior plan

Kids with ADD/ADHD can influence proper classroom behavior. However, they need structure and clear expectations to keep their signs and symptoms in check. As a parent, you can assist by developing a routine prepare for your youngster-- and also adhering to it. Whatever sort of habits plan you decide to execute, grow it in close collaboration with your child's instructor as well as your kid.

Children with a focus shortage problem respond best to details goals and also everyday positive reinforcement-- as well as valuable benefits. Yes, you may have to hang a carrot on a stay with inspiring your kid to act much better in the course. Produce a plan that includes small incentives for small success and more significant benefits for more massive accomplishments.

Tips for managing ADHD symptoms at college

ADHD impacts each kid's mind in different ways so that each instance can look entirely various in the classroom. Kids with ADHD exhibit a variety of signs and symptoms: some seem to bounce bizarre, some vision frequently, and also others can not appear to follow the guidelines.

As a parent, you can assist your child with ADHD to reduce any kind of or every one of these sorts of actions. It is essential to comprehend just how interest shortage disorder impacts different children's activities so that you can select the proper methods for dealing with the problem. There is a range of relatively uncomplicated approaches you and your child's teacher can require to most exceptional take care of the signs of ADHD-- and put your kid when traveling to college success.

Handling distractibility

Child classroom looking up Students with ADHD might end up being so quickly distracted by noises, passersby, or their thoughts that they frequently miss out on vital class details. These children have difficulty staying focused on jobs that call for sustained mental effort. They may seem as if they're listening to you, yet something gets in the way of their capacity to preserve the details.

Assisting children who sidetrack easily includes physical positioning, raised motion, and also damaging long stretches of infiltrating much shorter pieces.

Seat the child with ADHD away from windows and doors. Put family pets in another room or an edge while the trainee is functioning.

Alternative seated activities with those that enable the child to relocate their body around the space. Whenever feasible, integrate physical movement right into lessons.

Compose vital information down where the child can conveniently review and reference it. Remind the pupil where the data is located.

Split massive projects into smaller ones, and also enable children constant breaks.

Lowering interrupting

Kids with interest shortage problem might deal with managing their impulses, so they typically speak up of turn. In the class or the house, they call out or comment while others are speaking. Their outbursts may encounter as aggressive and even rude, creating social troubles also. The self-esteem of children with ADHD is frequently reasonably fragile, so directing this concern out in course or before family members doesn't help the issue-- and also may even make problems worse.

Fixing the disruptions of youngsters with ADHD must be done very carefully so that the kid's self-worth is preserved, particularly before others. Establish a "secret language" with the child with ADHD. You can use discreet gestures or words you have formerly agreed upon to allow the kid to know they are disrupting. Praise the child for interruption-free discussions.

Managing impulsivity

Kids with ADHD may act before thinking, developing challenging social situations, along with problems in the classroom. Children who have difficulty with impulse control might come off as aggressive or unruly. This is probably the most turbulent symptom of ADHD, specifically at the institution.

Techniques for handling impulsivity consist of habits plans, the prompt method for infractions, and a procedure for offering youngsters with ADHD a feeling of control over their day.

Make sure a written habits strategy is near the trainee. You can also tape it to the wall surface or the kid's work desk.

Give consequences instantly, complying with wrongdoing. Specify in your description, making sure the youngster recognizes how they misbehaved.

Identify good behavior out loud. Be specific in your appreciation, seeing to it the youngster knows what they did right.

Compose the routine for the day on the board or on a paper as well as cross off each thing as it is finished.

Youngsters with impulse problems might acquire a sense of control and feel calmer when they recognize what to anticipate.

Handling fidgeting as well as attention deficit disorder

Students with ADHD frequent, constant physical movement. It might appear like a battle for these children to stay in their seats. Children with ADD/ADHD might leap, kick, twist, fidget as well as or else relocate ways that make them difficult to teach.

Strategies for combating hyperactivity include creative means to allow the youngster with ADHD to move in proper methods at proper times. Releasing power in this manner may make it much easier for the youngster to keep their bodies calmer during work time.

Ask youngsters with ADHD to run a duty or complete a task for you, even if it just suggests strolling across the room to develop pencils or place meals away.

Urge a kid with ADHD to play a sporting activity-- or a minimum of run about before and after institution-- and also make sure the kid never misses out on recess or P.E.

Provide a tension round, tiny toy, or one more item for the child to squeeze or play with discreetly at their seat.

Restriction screen time in favor of time for motion.

Handling difficulty following directions

Difficulty adhering to instructions is a hallmark issue for numerous children with ADHD. These youngsters might resemble they understand as well as may even make a note of trends, yet after that aren't able to follow them as asked. In some cases, these trainees miss-steps as well as turn in an insufficient job, or misconstrue a task altogether and also wind up doing another thing entirely.

Helping kids with ADHD comply with directions means taking steps to break down and reinforce the steps associated with your guidelines, and also redirecting when essential. Try maintaining your courses extremely quick, allowing the youngster to complete one action and after that, return to find out what they ought to do next. If the youngster leaves the track, provide a tranquil suggestion, redirecting in a calm yet firm voice. Whenever possible, compose instructions down in a bold pen or colored chalk on a blackboard.

Tips for making finding out fun

Mommy helping a kid with homework One positive way to maintain your child's interest concentrated on discovering is to make the process enjoyable. Using physical activity in a lesson, attaching dry facts to fascinating trivia, or developing silly songs that make information much more comfortable to remember can aid your child delight in learning and even decrease the symptoms of ADHD.

Assisting youngsters with ADHD delight in math

Youngsters who have an interest deficiency problem tend to assume in a "concrete" fashion. They were typically such as to hold, touch, or take part in experience to learn something brand-new. By utilizing video games as well as objects to show mathematical concepts, you can reveal your youngster that math can be purposeful-- and also fun.

Play video games.

Use flash memory cards, dice, or dominoes to make numbers fun. Or merely utilize your fingers and toes, putting them in or shaking them when you add or deduct.

Attract pictures.

Specifically, for word troubles, illustrations can help kids better recognize mathematical principles. If words problem claims, there are twelve autos, help your youngster draw them from the guiding wheel to the trunk.

Create foolish acronyms. To bear in mind the order of operations, as an example, make up a track or expression that uses the initial letter of each procedure in the proper order.

Helping youngsters with ADHD enjoy reading

There are numerous means to make reading amazing, even if the skill itself often tends to present a battle for children with ADHD. Bear in mind that analysis at its a lot of fundamental level includes stories and interesting details-- which all kids delight in.

Read to youngsters. Make checking out relaxing, quality time with you.

Make predictions or "bets." Frequently ask the kid what they assume could occur next. Design prediction: "The lady in the story seems rather take on-- I bet she's most likely to try to conserve her household."

Act out the story. Let the youngster select their character and also designate you one. Use funny voices as well as outfits to bring it to life.

Exactly how does your child like to learn?

When children are given information in such a way that makes it very easy for them to absorb, learning is a lot of extra fun. If you recognize just how your child with ADHD learns best, you can develop delightful lessons that pack an informational strike.

Acoustic learners learn best by talking as well as listening. Have these kids recite facts to a favored track. Let them pretend they get on a radio show and also deal with others typically.

Visual students learn best with analysis or monitoring. Let them enjoy with various fonts on the computer system and also use tinted flashcards to examine. Enable them to write or attract their ideas theoretically.

Responsive learners learn best through physical touch or movement as part of a lesson. For these trainees, provide jellybeans for counters as well as outfits for acting out components of literature or history. Allow them to make use of clay and make collections.

Tips for understanding research

Certain, youngsters might globally dread it-- however, for moms and dad of a youngster with ADHD, research is a gold possibility. Academic work done outside the class offers you as the moms and dad with an opportunity to straight sustain your youngster. It's time you can help your youngster prosper at the institution where you both feel most comfortable: your living-room.

With your support, youngsters with ADHD can utilize research time not just for mathematics troubles or creating essays, but additionally for practicing the business and also research study skills they require to flourish in the class.

Aiding a youngster with ADHD get arranged

When it pertains to the company, it can assist in getting a fresh start. Also, if it's not the begin of the school year, go patronizing your child and select institution products that include folders, a three-ring binder, and also color-coded dividers. Assist the child to submit their papers right into this brand-new system.

Establish a research folder for finished research and also arrange loose papers by color-coding folders. Program your youngster how to file suitably.

Aid your kid to organize their belongings every day, including knapsack, folders, as well as even pockets.

If possible, maintain an additional set of textbooks as well as various other materials in the house.

Assist your youngster in discovering to make as well as use checklists, crossing products off as they accomplish them.

Assisting a kid with ADHD obtain research done on time

Recognizing concepts as well as receiving arranged are two activities in the right direction. Still, research also has to be completed in a single evening-- and kipped down on time. Help a youngster with ADHD to the finish line with techniques that supply constant structure.

Select a particular time and area for research that is as free as possible of clutter, family pets, as well as tv.

Enable the child breaks as typically as every 10 to twenty minutes.

Educate a far better understanding of the passage of time: use an analog clock as well as timers to monitor homework efficiency.

Establish a homework procedure at college: develop a place where the pupil can quickly discover their finished homework and also select a consistent time to hand in work to the teacher.

Other means to aid your kid with research

Encourage workout as well as sleep. Physical activity improves focus as well as advertises mind development. Significantly for youngsters with ADHD, it also leads to better rest, which consequently can decrease the ADHD signs and symptoms.

Help your child eat. Setting up regular healthy dishes and snacks while cutting back on junk and sugary foods can assist manage signs and symptoms of ADHD.

Deal with on your own, so you're far better able to take care of your child. Do not disregard your demands. Try to consume right, exercise, get sufficient rest, handle stress, and seek in-person assistance from family and friends.

TRIGGER FOODS FOR ADHD

Managing ADHD: 15 Foods to Avoid

ADHD, additionally known as Attention Deficit Hyperactivity Disorder, is a type of behavioral problem mostly seen in children. This disorder is identified by restlessness, inattentiveness, difficulty focusing, high degrees of undistinct energy, and impulsive actions. While a correct diet plan can not heal ADHD, people that follow specific dietary standards can benefit from eating effectively.

ADHD Medications

Many professionals think consuming certain foods can cause ADHD signs in individuals, particularly children, so it's important to avoid specific foods thought to stimulate a reaction.

If you or a person you love struggles with ADHD, try avoiding these 15 foods. Getting rid of (or firmly lowering) these foods from your diet can assist handle the symptoms of ADHD.

1. Ice Cream

Dairy items, such as ice cream, can set off ADHD in Individuals that are oversensitive to milk items. Somebody who is sensitive to dairy items might feel weary, both as well as psychologically, after eating foods such as gelato. Because of this, it's finest to prevent this chilly reward-- although it may seem like a great concept at the time.

2. Yogurt

Similar to ice cream, yogurt is a milk item that has been known to stimulate flare-ups in individuals with ADHD. Removing these types of products (milk items) entirely from your diet for a couple of weeks will undoubtedly assist in seeing whether they are a cause for ADHD. If dairy items activate your ADHD, think about changing them for foods made with soy instead.

3. Sugar

Professionals say a diet high in sugar can stimulate a flare in ADHD patients. Numerous experts think that the sugar strips your body of the vitamins, enzymes, and also minerals called for to assist support your mood.

4. Coffee

This might be a difficult one for numerous people to surrender, considering coffee is such a popular beverage. Lots of people count on coffee for an energetic start to their mornings. However, coffee contains a substantial quantity of high levels of caffeine, which-- an all-natural energizer understood to activate ADHD symptoms. If your symptoms get worse after drinking coffee, you can attempt drinking herbal teas or decaffeinated coffee instead.

5. Swordfish

Fish high in mercury, such as swordfish, have been recognized to cause ADHD signs and symptoms. The heavy steel (mercury) discovered in this kind of fish can reduce one's capability to concentrate and also hinder focus in many individuals. If you find out your symptoms getting worse after eating this kind of fish, select fish with reduced mercury levels such as shrimp, lobster or salmon.

6. Cheese

One more dairy food to stay clear of when attempting to prevent stimulating ADHD signs is cheese (especially cow's cheese). Similar to yogurt and ice cream, getting rid of cheese from your diet plan for 6 to eight weeks will assist in determining whether it's the cause for your flare-ups. If you observe your symptoms are extra manageable when you're not eating cheese (or various other cow dairy items), think about switching over to a lactose-free or cow dairy products free diet (i.e., eat goat's cheese rather).

7. Chocolate

Chocolate, like coffee, consists of a significant amount of caffeine. High levels of caffeine have been known to trigger ADHD signs and also can make signs even worse if you select not to eliminate it from your diet plan. If you notice, your symptoms worsen after consuming chocolaDiabetes-Friendly Thanksgiving Recipes.

8. Pop

Pop has human-made shades and flavoring, which several experts think can trigger signs in individuals with ADHD. In addition to human-made shades and flavoring, numerous stands out also have higher degrees of caffeine, which-- as explained formerly-- can activate ADHD signs and symptoms also. It's finest to avoid soda and go with a natural drink (homemade smoothies are incredible) instead.

9. Frozen Pizza

Icy pizzas are stuffed packed with synthetic shades as well as flavors, much like pop. The ingredients utilized to aid boost these types of products can raise attention deficit disorder and also decrease concentration in individuals with this condition. If you like consuming pizza, take into consideration making one from the ground up on your own. In this manner, you'll know every one of the active ingredients made use of are healthy and balanced and also natural

10. Corn

Yellow vegetables, such as corn, are known to trigger responses in people with ADHD. It is suggested that you avoid eating these types of veggies to help regulate your signs and symptoms. If you wish to eat wellness, opt for various other vegetables like spinach, peppers or tomatoes

11. Chips

It's virtually a considered that chips would be on this list. A lot of convenience food must be prevented to assist handle this type of problem. Microchips are also high in fabricated shades as well as a flavoring, making them a poor choice for individuals trying to find an ADHD bland diet. If you like snacking, take into consideration consuming healthy and balanced vegetables to suppress your cravings, instead of fast food like chips and delicious chocolate.

12. Squash

Squash is one more yellow food to avoid when managing ADHD. For the same factors as corn, squash has been recognized to create flare-ups. Not all yellow foods misbehave for people with ADHD-- bananas are all right since the real banana is white. Only the peel of the bananas is yellow, as well as you don't eat the yellow component anyways. As we pointed out earlier, select healthy (perhaps natural) veggies instead of yellow ones.

13. Fruit Juice

Many fruit juices are loaded with artificial shades and tastes. You need to avoid alcohol consumption fruit juices unless they are 100 percent natural without artificial coloring or flavor. Consider making a delicious healthy smoothie with fresh, organic fruits you've bought from the grocery store as opposed to boxed juice that's undesirable for several factors.

14. Junk food

Fast Food gets on the top of most "Do Not Eat" checklists, and this list is no exception. The fried foods found in the majority of fast food dishes are unbelievably unhealthy and the active ingredients have been recognized to cause an increase in ADHD symptoms. People seeking to handle their signs and symptoms need to stay clear of fast food entirely as well as select making dinner on your own.

15. Red Meat

Red meat has been understood to create an increase of symptoms for ADHD patients, experts state. Reducing your red meat intake (not necessarily eradicating it) may verify terrific benefits when it comes to controlling your ADHD. As pointed out previously, going with much healthier choices like salmon or shrimp will undoubtedly aid in keeping your symptoms managed so you can maintain a more active, better life.

THE IMPORTANCE OF KEEPING AN ADHD JOURNAL

Coping with a mental wellness problem can be difficult, yet journaling might aid. Journaling can help you to handle anxiety, anxiousness, depression, and also bipolar illness. Also, you can utilize your journal to assist you in improving your routines as well as behaviors. To begin journaling, select a convenient time to compose each day as well as obstacle yourself to write whatever involves your mind for 20 minutes. Utilize your journal to process your feelings or deal with your self-improvement goals.

Determine if you intend to maintain a paper journal or an electronic journal.

Usually, writing by hand aids, you refine your ideas much better. Nonetheless, it's ideal to choose whichever style is most convenient for you. Choose a paper journal if you delight in composing by hand, or utilize a word processor if you prefer to type.

A paper journal will make it less complicated to get imaginative with your entries if you're interested in including art in your journal.

You may be able to include in your digital journal from any device if you use Google Docs. Download Google Docs free of charge from the app store. After that, produce as well as modify records on any device that has Google Docs.

Write in your journal daily to get one of the most benefits.

It's essential to create a practice if you intend to use your journal to boost your mental wellness. Pick a time when it's convenient for you to write after that challenge yourself to create daily. Arrange your journaling time right into your day like any various other essential consultation.

You might compose in your journal every early morning when you wake up, during your lunch hr, or directly before bed.

If you commute by bus or train, use that time to write in your journal.

Set a timer for 20 minutes as well as attempt to create until it goes off.

When you first start journaling, provide yourself a brief home window of time to do it, so it does not feel overwhelming. Begin with 20 mins, but feel free to readjust the time to fit your requirements better. While the timer is going, write down or type any words that stand out into your head.

While the goal is to discuss your thoughts or stress factors, do not bother with that right now. It's all right to compose points like, "I don't understand what to claim," "This feels silly," or "I can't think of anything today." If you keep going, you'll begin to discover your internal thoughts.

Pointer: It's okay to keep creating after the timer goes off. The objective of the timer is to assist you in feeling like there's structure to your journaling practice, which may help you start much more conveniently.

Don't bother with punctuation or grammar.

Your journal is for you, so it doesn't matter if you make use of appropriate sentences or spell words appropriately. Let your thoughts circulation openly with no self-editing.

If your grammar mistakes honestly bother you, it's alright to return and correct them at a later time. Nevertheless, this isn't needed.

Get creative with your formatting if you do not know, such as writing in sentences.

You can still get the benefits of journaling even if you hate writing or can't determine what to state. Don't bother with drawing up sentences or paragraphs. Try various ways of formatting entrances until you find one that works for you. Below are some ways you might express on your own:

Make a list.

Create a rhyme or song.

Include photos to reveal precisely how you feel or what's on your mind.

Write a letter to somebody.

Create a tale with you as a significant personality.

Usage sentence stems from your specialist or online. These could include, "I feel most dismayed when ...," "I feel my ideal when ... " or "I'm most anxious concerning ...".

Make A Bullet Journal.

Make Your Journal A Judgment-Free Zone.

Provide on your authorization to compose whatever you're feeling without policing your ideas. Do not attach negative emotions like regret or shame to what you. You have every right to your thoughts and also feelings, and your journaling technique is your method helps them be as healthy and balanced as possible. Do not evaluate yourself for making this excellent step towards fixing your internal problems.

You may feel guilty for raving out over something that took place in your day. Do not judge on your own for obtaining distressed since that's an entirely reasonable reaction. Instead, pat yourself on the back for working through those ideas in your journal.

Managing Thoughts and also Feelings.

Express whatever is on your mind when you sit down to write.

The most effective means to use journaling to refine your ideas and feelings is to blog about what's going on in your life that day. Discuss what's happened to you, how you feel about points, as well as any worries that you have. Keep creating up until your timer goes off, or you feel much better.

You might create something like, "Today, I felt unfortunate since it was drizzling all the time. I assume the weather condition influences my state of mind. I question how I can help myself feel better on gloomy days.".

Compose in a stream of aware when you're not sure what you're feeling.

Occasionally it's tough to understand what's really on your mind, which's fine! To create a stream of aware, take-down any words that enter your account, even if they don't make good sense. Don't worry about spelling or syntax. Keep creating up until you recognize a central point or motif arising, which will certainly inform you exactly how you feel.

As an example, a stream of mindful entrance might resemble this: "Sitting right here simply not recognizing what to state it's been a long day as well as I'm exhausted but I can't identify why I feel down today and I believe it's since points have not been going my means so possibly I need to alter something however what can I alter.".

Release unfavorable emotions like temper, sadness, and also envy.

Every person manages setbacks and also disputes, and even occasionally, it's challenging to resolve the intense negative feelings that these scenarios activate. Your journal is a device that you can use to process these emotions and number out your next steps. Draw up a tirade or issue about every little thing that's going wrong. Compose a letter to the individual who hurt you yet don't send it.

Create something like, "I can not think Alex did not give me the help she guaranteed.

I assumed I might depend on her. I wanted to chew out her until my face transforms blue. However, I do not want a bunch of drama from my mother."

Suggestion: Writing down how you feel can aid you to calm down as well as locate words you need to communicate your feelings to others. After you reveal on your own in your journal, examine what you've written and also determine what you require to do besides attend to the problem.

Track your moods every day to help you recognize your triggers.

Recording your mood in your journal entries aids you in acknowledging patterns that might lead you to your triggers. Document just how you felt throughout the day, either before or after your journal access. Additionally, rate your mood on a numerical scale. Look back over your state of mind to see what assists you feel terrific and what causes a low state of mind.

This can aid you in making favorable changes to improve your mood in total.

You might write your state of mind in a word or make use of a symbol. Possible moods may consist of "satisfied," "depressing," "stressed out," "uncaring," or "mad." You could rate your moods on a scale of 1-5, with 1 being light as well as five being extreme. Create something like "Depressed.".

Assess your entrances to help you much better comprehend your feelings.

To obtain the most out of your journaling behavior, return, and also re-read what you've created at a later time. Think about what you claimed and just how you must have been feeling. Use this to assist you in making better choices for yourself in the future. Additionally, it might aid you to reframe your thoughts so you can think in different ways regarding things in the future.

If you're undergoing a crisis, you might re-read your entry right after you wrote it or later that same day.

If you intend to enhance your general mental wellness, evaluate your posts after 3-4 months.

Using Your Journal for Self-Improvement.

Track your progression towards objectives, excellent habits, as well as positive behaviors. Use your journal to establish individual goals and also work toward favorable habits or behaviors you want to integrate into your life. Tape the actions you're taking toward your objectives and check your development. Besides, make a note of or mark off when you engage in your good practices or habits.

You might maintain a web page in your journal to track your development on your goal. Compose an action plan, paper when you work on the objective, and check off each action.

If your goal was to meditate daily, you might block off time to practice meditation in your timetable as well as download a meditation application. After that, keep track of how frequently you meditate, the length of time your sessions last, and also the benefits you feel after reflection.

Offer on your own a sticker label or checkmark on days you work towards your goal or brand-new habits. As an example, provide yourself a face sticker label each time you do self-care, a checkmark for each glass of water you consume, or a star each day you prepare a dish in your home.

File your symptoms if you're dealing with a mental disease.

Tracking your signs and symptoms can help you identify if you're making progress or which treatments work best for you. Write down the signs you're experiencing at the top or base of your journal entrance for that day. Rate the extent of your symptoms on a mathematical range so you can better recognize them. Compare the symptoms you're experiencing with what was happening in your life that day to help you seek patterns.

You might create, "Today, I feel anxious as well as uncertain with the numbers representing the seriousness of your symptoms.

If you're on medicine, keep an eye on when you take it to see if that has any influence on your signs.

Tape proof for or versus your ideas concerning yourself.

You likely have a mix of favorable as well as adverse beliefs about yourself. Sometimes, a lot of unfavorable ideas can include in your clinical depression and stress and anxiety, even though they may not be accurate. When you have a negative thought regarding on your own, document the proof you have to both think and also disbelieve that thought. Use this technique to help you view on your own in a more favorable light.

Let's state you think that you're foolish. You could detail examples of times you've claimed something clever, topics that you're specifically knowledgeable concerning, and also any type of education that you've completed. From there, you may state, "I'm actually wise when it comes to background and aiding people organize their things.".

Make a benefits and drawbacks list if you have a big decision to make.

Huge choices are always hard, however in some cases they can really feel a lot more overwhelming if you're taking care of a mental illness. Your journal can aid you figure out what to do. Draw the line down the facility of your page, then list the pros of a choice on the left side and the disadvantages on the best side. Develop a checklist for each option you're thinking about, then choose the choice that profits you the most.

You may just require to make 1 benefits and drawbacks checklist to assist you choose.

For instance, let's state you're determining whether or not to obtain an emotional support animal. Pros might consist of, "Having convenience," "Never feeling alone," and "Feeling satisfied when I see my buddy." Cons could consist of, "Need to clean up after it," and "Have to do paperwork.".

It's practical to make multiple listings if you have a number of various choices. As an example, you may make multiple lists if you're determining which treatment choice to attempt.

Exactly how To Keep A Parenting Journal

Many people maintain parenting journals either to keep records for safekeeping situations or to preserve memories for their family members. While protection journals should be objective documents, journals for families need to capture the emotions related to memories. When maintaining either type of journal, however, you will wish to compose as usually as feasible and also document as much as you can.

Compose Consistently.

When keeping a wardship journal, it's critical that you write in it on a regular basis in order to make it as trusted as well as authoritative as feasible. By taping info each day-- or perhaps several times a day-- you can be certain that what you are creating is as accurate as well as beneficial as feasible.

If you write much less commonly, you run the risk of being unclear and nonspecific. You may likewise just fail to remember information you meant to tape-record.

Keep Objective.

While custody circumstances can be difficult, you require to remain as objective as possible in your custody journal. This is not an opportunity to vent your frustrations or demonize the various other parent. Journal entrances that are certainly psychological will be less useful in a legal setting.

If you feel like you need to overcome your emotions by composing them down, attempt maintaining a totally separate journal or diary. That way you can express yourself without jeopardizing your custody journal.

An instance of suitable objective writing is: "John picked up our youngster at 4:00. The scheduled pick-up time was 3:00." An unacceptable account of the exact same event would state something like: "John was late once more today, like normal. He is so reckless and also a bad parent."

Keep a thorough document of your child's routine.

Your attorney will certainly require as many facts concerning your youngster's life as well as wellness as possible. To aid your attorney, keep a detailed log of what your youngster does daily. You can keep in mind things like medical visits, extracurricular activities, time spent with buddies, and so forth. The more info you can provide the far better.

Note your role in your child's life.

Videotape when you drive them to appointments, make them meals, assist with research, and anything else you do to assist increase them. You will want to ensure that your custody journal shows the crucial duty you play in your kid's life.

Keep notes on all communication with the other moms and dad.

You must make a note of each time you interact with the various other parent, whether in person or online. Make a note of details regarding the moment, day, approach, as well as length of the communication. You must additionally note the topic of the discussion, but you do not have to do so in fantastic detail.

Consist of screenshots or printouts of the communication, if possible.

Track the various other parent's obligations.

You will undoubtedly wish to maintain detailed notes regarding exactly how well the various other moms and dad fulfill their obligations. Make a note of pick-up times and drop-off times. If the other moms and dad start to shirk responsibilities, take down each instance. Remember to stay objective, though.

To see to it, you continue to be objective; you ought to also keep in mind each time the other moms and dad meet responsibilities. For example, you can document something like: "Sarah took our youngster to the dentist today as well as brought her back home on time."

Videotape what your youngster states about the other parent.

Exactly how your kid feels concerning the other moms and dad is extremely important, so you need to attempt to record that in addition to you can. Among the most effective methods to do this is to keep notes concerning the essential things your child claims about the other parent, using straight quotes. You do not need to require your youngster to say features of the other parent, yet compose it down whenever the subject shows up.

As always, tape the excellent along with the bad to see to it you're staying goal.

Concentrate on the child's behavior as opposed to your very own impacts. As opposed to claiming, "John is emotional as well as sad today," create, "John frowned all morning. He cried to 15 mins at 1 pm."

Track your kid's mood and also habits.

To track exactly how your guardianship scenario is affecting a child's emotional health and wellness, you ought to take comprehensive notes concerning exactly how they are behaving. If a child acts in different ways than usual after being around the various other moms and dads, you can take down that.

By keeping track of your kid's mental health in this way, you can also make sure that you concern a custody arrangement that is ideal for them.

Videotape your kid's performance in college.

You can likewise monitor your kid's well-being by tape-recording their performance in the institution as well as any extracurricular activities. You wish to be able to determine if your custodianship plan is impacting your youngster's capability to succeed in college whatsoever.

You need to keep in mind test ratings and progress reports, whether they are excellent or bad.

If your child is having behavioral problems in school, track these as well.

Maintaining a Journal for Family Memories

Choose a writing technique you like.

You can choose to write your parenting journal in whatever way you would certainly such as. You can write with a pen or book a physical journal or create digitally on your laptop computer or tablet. One of the most important things is to select an approach that will enable you to write as frequently and also conveniently as feasible. Just like a custody journal, you need to write as commonly as you can. It ensures that you can be as particular as well as detailed as possible.

Begin journaling when you know you are expecting.

If you're creating because you want to record your youngster's life and also share your parenting journey with your family members, you must begin as quickly as you can. The day you figure out you're expecting can be an excellent time to start a parenting journal. In this manner, you will have the ability to tape as a number of your thoughts and experiences as feasible.

Track milestones.

A parenting journal is a beautiful location to tape landmarks in your child's life, such as when they take their first step or claim their very first word. Whenever anything that appears considerable happens to your child, keep in mind the occasion as well as when it occurred in your parenting journal.

You can determine what counts as a milestone, however, you desire. Even if something seems relatively little, you ought to videotape it if it's essential to you as well as your child.

You can likewise use a child publication instead of an empty journal. Child books are mostly empty yet are gotten into sections devoted to developmental milestones, such as losing teeth.

Include images of significant moments in a kid's life to assist maintain the memories even much better.

Express your feelings.

Do not merely videotape what took place during the day; define precisely how you feel concerning it. You will undoubtedly want your parenting journal to protect not just facts; however, the emotional experiences of your family members. When you blog about something charming your kid has done, describe just how it made you feel. It will undoubtedly make your journal a touching record a period in your family's life that passes promptly.

Someday, your children will read this journal and will undoubtedly wonder to learn about what you were like currently. The even more details regarding your mood you can give, the extra you can satisfy that inquisitiveness.

Focus on the favorable.

You don't require to stay away from unfavorable topics entirely, yet you do not wish to dwell on them. Being as well negative could injure the sensations of your youngster if you wind up sharing the journal with them. You intend to make sure you're focusing mainly on the happy moments that you as well as your kid, share.

Show your journal to your child when they're ready.

Among the objectives of a family, parenting journal is to be able to utilize it to reveal your children what their very early life was like, as they will have no memories of it. Whenever you feel your kid prepares to see what you've created and recorded, you can share it with them.

If you've written a great deal concerning on your own as well as your emotions, you may want to wait up until your child is older.

SIMPLE HINTS AND POINTERS FOR AVOIDING MELTDOWN

1. Pinpoint the source.

Psychotherapist Stephanie Sarkis, Ph.D., recommended looking "at what might be causing your child's actions." When you can locate the resource of the habits, she said, you can make strides towards changing it.

Knowing what triggers your youngster, Matlen stated, can assist you in defusing their tantrum as very early as possible. For instance, is your youngster starving? Are they sleep-deprived? Are they experiencing stable emotions? As soon as you pinpoint the underlying problem, attempt to solve it, she stated.

Additionally is an excellent device for protecting against temper tantrums. If your kid can not manage the overstimulating environment of a neighborhood fair, don't take them, Matlen said.

2. Explain the consequences in advance.

Before a temper tantrum ever before starts, Matlen recommended talking with your kid regarding the unfavorable consequences of negative behaviors. She provided this instance: "If you yell as well as weep when I switch off the TV, you won't be able to enjoy it later today."

Matlen took this strategy when her little girl was five years old. She tended to have temper tantrums when she did not get a brand-new plaything at the shop. "Before our next outing, I informed her that if she had an outburst, I would choose her up and take her house. No playthings and also no more brows through to the store for a very long time."

Her daughter still had a meltdown. However, as opposed to obtaining angry or frustrated, Matlen picked up her child as well as took her to the cars and truck. She drove residence without stating a word as well as it never occurred once more.

" This, of course, might not work for all youngsters, yet it's an example of intending in advance and also having an outcome that every person comprehends."

3. Talk with your kid, as well as urge them to debate.

Talk smoothly as well as quietly to your child, and recognize their feelings, Matlen stated. Doing so helps your child feel listened to, Sarkis claimed.

According to Matlen, you could state, "I recognize you're angry that I won't buy you that plaything today. It feels frustrating and it makes you seem like taking off inside, does not it?"

Then, urge your child to express their feelings, also: "I 'd be distressed also if I could not obtain what I wanted right now-- let's talk about why this is so vital to you so you can help me to understand."

4. Sidetrack your youngster.

For younger children, distraction might work, Matlen stated. "Talk concerning something completely various, like exactly how thrilled you are to enjoy the TELEVISION program you intended when you all get home."

5. Give them a break.

" Sometimes, absolutely nothing seems to work, though, and also a child will certainly not quit regardless of what you attempt," Matlen said. When that occurs, comfortably clarify that they'll need to visit their area. They can appear after they've calmed down. It is an effective way to learn self-soothing actions, she stated. As a result of that, it's crucial to maintain items that advertise healthy copings, such as a teddy bear or fidget playthings, she added.

6. Overlook the tantrum.

" Sometimes the very best response to an outburst is no response," said Sarkis, writer of numerous publications on ADHD, consisting of Making the Grade with ADD: A Student's Guide to Succeeding in College with Attention Deficit Disorder. That's because "even unfavorable interest is the focus, as well as it provides a 'reward' for the actions." So not offering your youngster a "target market" could assist in decreasing the size of the outburst.

If your child has an outburst in the center of the shop-- and it's not crowded-- let them have the tantrum, Sarkis said. "You might get looks from others. It's ALRIGHT. Just bear in mind that not paying attention to the habits assists extinguish it."

7. Provide tips.

According to both experts, kids with ADHD have a hard time with shifts. They can have a meltdown when it's time to leave the play area or stop playing their videogame to have dinner, Matlen claimed. "Things that are enjoyable are hard to quit, especially when the transition is into a task they might not appreciate."

This is when pointers are essential. For example, remind your kid at 30, 15, 10, and 5-minute intervals that supper prepares, Matlen claimed. Additionally, establish appropriate consequences if they do not conform, such as not playing videogames after dinner, or playing them for 15 minutes as opposed to 30 following time, she stated. (Or just restriction videogames before dinner entirely, she claimed.).

Matlen provided this instance of what to claim to your child: "I recognize it's difficult for you to stop playing your PlayStation when it's time for supper. I will provide you reminders so that you can wind down. Nevertheless, having a temper tantrum is not acceptable, so if that happens, you will certainly (fill in the space).".

8. Commend your kid when they do show self-control.

" Parents require to catch their kids being great far more than they capture them being 'bad,'" Sarkis stated. "Children with ADHD react well to positive support." And also, "whatever you focus on grows," she added.

According to Matlen, rather than saying, "You are such an excellent young boy for not having a meltdown when I said no to ice cream," a much better response would undoubtedly be, "You have to have truly felt pleased with on your own that you did not have a tantrum when you saw that we were out of cookies-- excellent job!".

9. Avoid corporal penalties.

It's a typical response to snap when a moms and dad sees his/her kid flat out on the flooring lashing out, kicking as well as screaming," Matlen said. You might grab your youngster or perhaps spank them. However, this only gas the negative situation as well as every person's feelings, she claimed. "Corporal penalty might soothe the behavior temporarily-- though normally, it just raises the negative behavior-- yet it additionally establishes the tone that it's OKAY to hit people when you're mad." Also, a youngster requires to "get himself in control.".

Taking care of tantrums is difficult. By planning, staying calm as well as applying particular methods, you can appease them. And also, if the temper tantrum does not go silent, try to ride it out.

Precisely How To Prevent After-School Meltdowns

As moms and dad, you may observe that your youngster leaves for school packed with joy and also gets back under a dark cloud. They may blast you, toss a tantrum, or have a full meltdown after college. It is called "after-school restraint collapse," and it occurs because the school can be mentally draining. Therefore, they may be in a weary, irritated state of mind when they obtain a house. You can prevent after-school crises by producing a regular for your child to adhere to and also by maintaining them calm as quickly as they enter the door. If your youngster has an after-school meltdown, you need steps to moderate the situation as well as convenience them.

Identify that troubles during college can cause bottled-up anxiety.

The institution can be a challenging experience for some children. Handling their emotions and impulses is hard work.

They might keep their feelings shut in until they reach a place where they feel secure. (The excellent news is that your youngster does feel safe in your home, or they would not discharge their emotions.).

Understand variables that make some youngsters extra susceptible to meltdowns after college.

Age, perfectionism, and also impairments can cause children having a more difficult time dealing with the stress and anxiety of college.

Age plays a role in after-school disasters. More youthful children are less mentally resilient, as well as, therefore, more likely to thaw down. They are expected to grow out of these disasters.

Perfectionism can make a child seem like they need to be "best" at school.

Therefore, they may be an angel at the institution, only to break down in rips once they get home.

Impairments like dyslexia or autism can suggest that kids require added assistance at school, as well as they might not always get sufficient aid. They may also be rejected or criticized unfairly by peers or teachers.

Recognize that severe or regular after-school disasters might signify a much deeper issue.

If your child's meltdowns are unusually horrible or frequent, after that, it may suggest that points aren't okay at school. Your kid might be handling an issue like.

Bullying.

A mean instructor.

Frustrating schoolwork.

Too much stress to perform.

Stress and anxiety issues.

Lack of ample assistance for special needs (diagnosed or undiagnosed).

Speak up if you believe that something is seriously incorrect.

If your youngster's disasters look like they are abnormally regular or extreme, then that indicates that there can be an underlying issue. Do not wait it out. Instead, ask other people concerning what's going on.

Ask your youngster. What makes school hard? What is the hardest component of school? What are the various other youngsters like?

Ask other moms and dads.

Do their kids have similar disasters, or make your child's meltdowns sound means even worse than average?

Ask your youngster's teachers.

What takes place at college that could be creating so much anxiety? Exist in any social or academic troubles? Does your youngster seem to be having a problem with stress and anxiety administration?

Ask your child's pediatrician.

Are these crises normal for their age, or could the youngster be experiencing an emotional handicap?

Creating an After-School Routine.

Welcome your child with a smile, as well as no questions.

When your kid gets home from college, avoid annoying them with great deals of questions about their day or just how they feel. Conserve the concerns for a later time when they are resolved and also relaxed. Instead, greet them with a smile as well as a "welcome home" or a "great to have you back." Be cozy and also positive when they walk through the door so they begin to really feel much more loosened up as well as tranquil.

You can also try asking your youngster, "Do you intend to discuss your day now or later on?" They have the alternative to informing you about their day currently or at one more time. This will show them that you appreciate their day yet comprehend they may be bewildered and also require a long time to unwind before you speak.

Have treats or a meal ready for them.

Many youngsters get back from institutions hungry, as well as hunger integrated with irritability or fatigue can cause a tiff. Avoid a meltdown by providing them treats or a tiny dish right when they get home. You can likewise put some snacks out in a bowl in the kitchen area so they can access them on their own.

If the drive from the college to your home is a long one, bring a snack so your child can consume it on the playground or in the vehicle on the way home.

You may prepare healthy treats like cut-up fruit or a dish of nuts. You can also leave out crackers or chips for your youngster to snack on when they obtain home from college so they please their appetite yet not spoil their appetite for supper.

Let your child have some downtime alone.

You should additionally make downtime part of your child's after-school regimen, where they can take a break as well as have time to themselves. Giving your youngster an hr of downtime once they get to the house can aid them to relax and also release several of the anxiousness or tension of their college day.

You may offer your child an hour to themselves in their room where they can take place their computer, listen to music, or review.

Your youngster may likewise favor being active as a component of their downtime where they play a sporting activity outside or run about in the yard for an hour after college.

If your kid appears exhausted, supply a chance for them to take a nap.

Prepare your youngster for research or dinner.

As a component of your youngster's after-school routine, you need to additionally prepare your kid for homework at night as well as dinnertime. Provide a half an hour to an hr to themselves, and after that, remind them that they must start their homework in the next fifty percent hr to an hour. You also need to allow them to recognize what time dinner will be so they can plan for it. In this manner, they feel much less worried as well as can stay with a regular.

As an example, you may inform your youngster, "How regarding we do research in 30 mins together at the cooking area table?" or "Remember that dinner is in an hour, fine?".

Keeping Your Child Calm After School.

Establish a calm atmosphere for them.

An additional way you can prevent your child from having a meltdown when they get home from college is to create a residence atmosphere that is tranquil as well as kicking back for them. Prevent having great deals of mess everywhere in your house and also keep the noise degree down. Clean the common area and also laid out your child's plaything so they are simple to access when they get home from college.

You might also attempt to establish a tranquil setting for yourself as well, such as lighting candle lights, placing on relaxing music, and even doing a relaxing task before your child gets home. It could, after that, aid you set a calm tone for your youngster when they walk through the door.

Do enjoyable, involving activities with your child.

You can likewise keep your kid's spirits up when they get to the house by supplying to do some fun activities with them when they get home. Possibly you set up a craft location where you can attract and also repaint with each other. Or perhaps you bring out your kid's favored parlor game and also recommend you play around together. It can help your kid remain involved and also work off any adverse energy they are bringing home with them.

You may say to your youngster, "How concerning we get imaginative and do some crafts before homework?" or "Do you intend to play a board game before dinner?".

Enable them to play with brothers or sisters or buddies.

You ought to additionally urge your child to burn off any negative power from school by playing with brother or sisters or buddies. Possibly your youngster has a neighborhood good friend nearby that they like to run around with outside. Or probably your kid invites a close friend over to hang around in their space after school. Let them have good friends over so they can destress and also have fun.

For example, you may state to your youngster, "Do you want to invite a buddy over to play?" or "Would you such as to go have fun with your friend across the street?".

Recognize your kid's sensations.

If your youngster does have an after-school meltdown, you must be prepared for it and also handle it as necessary. Start by recognizing your youngster's feelings. They are likely feeling tired, stressed out, as well as inflamed. Comfort them that you understand they are exhausted from the institution and lashing out because they are worried. Doing this can aid to deescalate the situation and also allow them to recognize you get on their side.

For instance, you may state to your kid, "We're tired out from institution, aren't we?" or "You had a long day, didn't you? You're all set to have a snack and also relax.".

A visual sensations graph would undoubtedly be useful if your youngster is still finding out how to connect their feelings.

Separate your kid from others.

If there are various other kids in your home, you should have your kid transfer to a separate location, such as their bedroom. It will give them an area to cool down and also take a couple of deep breaths. Have them stay in their space for five to ten minutes, as this will certainly provide a chance to cool down as well as be on their very own.

Often, some alone time in a safe room like their room can assist them to unwind and release any tension from college.

It is likewise an excellent way to stay clear of distressing the other youngsters and help to maintain a calm area for everyone else in your household.

Offer your kid time and also the area to relax by themselves.

Instead of trying to fix your kid's issue for them or snap at them, let them calm down on their own. You might leave them with their toys or books as well as a tiny treat. After a few mins, they must calm down and come to be engaged in a plaything or their snack.

As soon as your child has cooled down as well as the meltdown has passed, you may then inquire concerning their day at the institution or ask if they 'd like to have fun with you. Involve with them just after they have relaxed.

DECREASING YOUR STRESS DEGREES ON ADHD -- IS IT POSSIBLE?

If you have ADHD, you might have difficulty with the company, listening abilities, as well as focusing. It can result in a lot of stress as well as frustration. It's all-natural to have a tough time when every day could seem like a fight.

Right here are some ways to aid manage your stress.

Practice deep breathing.

This strategy loads a one-two punch by reducing ADHD signs as well as reducing stress and anxiety. Finding out to use your breath to your advantage can aid you to boost leisure and also boost attention. Deep breathing jumpstarts your body's all-natural stress feedback, assisting you progressively end up being more secure. Right here's exactly how to do it.

Situate a place where you can be in peace for several minutes without disturbance. Sit down comfortably and also close your eyes. Breathe in genuinely and also gradually via your nose, ensuring that your stomach is expanding with each inhales. Release the air by exhaling through your mouth, noticing your stubborn belly deflating like a balloon. Repeat this exercise numerous times

Find out mindfulness.

It may appear not likely for a person with ADHD to successfully practice mindfulness. Still, the study shows it is really possible as well as likewise effective at decreasing signs and symptoms. Mindfulness is the practice of concentrating on the present moment, which can be a significant obstacle for individuals with ADHD. Researches show that mindfulness training can help improve focus. What's even more, mindfulness techniques are also efficient at minimizing stress and stress and anxiety.

To practice mindfulness, find a quiet location where you can sit comfortably for around 15 to 20 minutes without disturbances. Unwind your arm or legs. Shut your eyes and take a breath generally. Currently, start deep breathing, taking long, sluggish inhales in with your nose. Then, exhale slowly through your mouth. You can count emotionally as well as state "1." Repeat. Whenever you discover that your ideas have strayed, return your emphasis to your breath as well as restart your matter at one again.

Understanding mindfulness to get rid of ADHD on your own can be quite severe. Speak with your psychotherapist or mental wellness provider regarding completing a mindfulness training program under specialist supervision.

Relieve tension in your body.

If you are feeling stressed out, there are likely indications of stress in your body. Progressive muscular tissue relaxation instructs you exactly how to utilize your organization to lower pressure. This exercise can be included in a deep breathing practice for dual the advantage.

Do this workout in a quiet, secluded area. Lie down pleasantly on a couch or a bed. Relax your muscle mass as well as take several deep, cleansing breaths. Gradually relocate through each significant muscle team in your body, having and then launching the muscle mass.

Begin at your temple.

Scrunch up your forehead as well as curve your eyebrows for a couple of secs. Launch the stress and also discover how it feels when the pressure goes away. Transfer to the next muscular tissue team until you have completed your entire body. Once the exercise is completed, you should feel both emotionally and also literally relaxed.

Set up in time for play or relaxation.

Not having special times to look after yourself or locate satisfaction establishes you up for exhaustion at college or work. Make time weekly (or each day, if possible) to engage in a task that you locate pleasurably. It may consist of strolling on the beach, having fun with your pet dog, watching a preferred funny motion picture, or cooking cookies. Make time to do what you like typically.

Be patient with yourself. Don't beat yourself up.

Recognize that you are dealing with a severe mental condition in which you will undoubtedly make mistakes. If you hold on your own to the criterion of people without ADHD, you will always feel like a failure.

Instead, offer yourself a break and celebrate the small successes that you accomplish in a day. These may consist of getting to function or institution promptly or remembering to jot down your research or tasks listing.

Advocate on your own.

Being conscious of your needs as well as using your voice can help you lessen excess stress in the long haul. Successfully fighting ADHD and stress and anxiety call for that you end up being experienced about both problems and your constraints. When you know yourself as well as your demands, you are much better geared up to communicate those needs to others.

Educate on your own extensively regarding both ADHD and also stress and anxiety as well as know the signs and symptoms of each. Want to speak up at school or the workplace if you are being asked to carry out in a way that is tough for you as a result of these problems.

As an example, if you have trouble taking examinations within an arranged home window, you may need to consult with your school concerning obtaining test-taking lodgings. Increase your hand or draw your teacher aside and state, "Ms. Winters, it's stressful for me to complete my test in 45 minutes. Can you work with me to ensure that I do not feel so much anxiousness about taking examinations?"

Find out to identify and also stay clear of triggers.

You automatically really feel a lot more efficient in managing stress and anxiousness related to ADHD when you can acknowledge what's creating it. Fears, clutter, as well as still time are all potential triggers that

When you have determined your triggers, take a seat, and come up with options to ensure that you can prevent them completely. If idle time appears to set off anxiousness in you, it can be valuable to develop an everyday timetable that maintains you valid and active while consisting of a list of recreation activities you can do throughout your free time. In this way, you won't need to feel stressed out concerning downtime, you can merely take part in one of your set tasks throughout that time.

Get systems in position to counteract organizational concerns.

You may be against developing a regular, doing so can aid profoundly. Produce a feeling of structure in your life that aids you reduce stress and also decreases lack of organization.

As an example, you could invest some time each night getting prepared for the complying with day Lay out your clothes. Collect any essential files, such as kinds or projects.

You can likewise create a system for arranging documentation that has left hand as well as finishing homework. Talk to your institution psychotherapist, psychological health and wellness service providers, or educators to see if they can suggest any valuable systems for you to implement into day-to-day life.

Manage your time efficiently.

A person with ADHD may have trouble assessing time and handling target dates if you recognize that this is an obstacle for you, research methods to use to boost your time-management abilities.

These may consist of establishing timers that tell you when to quit one task as well as the move to an additional. Or, you may require to develop suggestions on your phone so that you do not forget crucial consultations or events. Recognize your restrictions as well as place steps in the position that aid you.

Take breaks when needed.

Stress can be developing as well as you did not also notice it. To effectively take care of anxiety, you need to have all-natural breaks into your day that enable you to see the tension and alleviate it before it places.

Every hour approximately, time out as well as take inventory of how your body feels. Exists stress present? Is your heart racing? Are you feeling overwhelmed? Are your ideas negative?

If you spot the signs of mounting stress, act, close your eyes and several full mins of deep breathing. Stretch your legs and go for a walk in nature. Call a buddy for a fast conversation. It's essential to discover when you're feeling stressed out as well as implement procedures to decrease it as necessary.

Following up with Treatment

Speak with your medical professional about using stimulants appropriately.

Although stimulant medications have shown to be highly effective in dealing with the signs of ADHD, this benefit does not come without expense. Energizers have the power to trigger or get worse existing stress and anxiety signs and symptoms.

Some medical professionals state that the stress and anxiety felt while taking stimulants takes place as the body adjusts to the medication, which symptoms should decrease in the coming days and weeks. All the same, your doctor can also recommend a non-stimulant in conjunction with a discerning serotonin reuptake prevention (SSRI) for people who can not tolerate stimulant drugs.

Another option is to take a drug to treat among the disorder (i.e., the ADHD or the anxiousness) and manage the various other with behavioral and lifestyle changes.

Attempt treatment if it aids.

Trying to deal with either ADHD or anxiousness with drugs only may not demonstrate optimal outcomes. Individuals must think about global lifestyle modifications in enhancement to various other specialist therapies, such as action therapy.

Behavior therapy is a treatment strategy helped with by a doctor, college psychotherapist, or various other psychological health and wellness providers to improve the more subtle signs and symptoms of ADHD. A structured program is developed that makes use of incentives and also consequences to boost abilities and remove unwanted behavior patterns.

Adjustment your diet plan as necessary.

There is no clear evidence that dietary and also dietary shortages create ADHD or anxiousness; there is evidence to show positive modifications can boost signs in both disorders. Foods that help the mind are helpful for individuals with ADHD.

These include a wealth of proteins discovered in meat, poultry, beans, nuts, as well as cheese. Eat much less straightforward carbohydrates like sugar, white flour, and white rice as well as even more complicated carbohydrates located in fruits, vegetables, and also whole grains. Foods with omega-3 fatty acids likewise help, such as salmon and also walnuts.

Nutritional supplements may likewise lower signs. Consider taking a 100% minerals and vitamin supplement daily.

Exercise frequently.

You might currently have received a suggestion to apply a regimen of exercise from your primary care medical professional. Regular exercise helps develop strong bones and also muscle mass. Nevertheless, along with physical fitness, exercise additionally assists the mind.

Neurotransmitters, select chemicals in mind, are created during exercise that can decrease inattention and also enhance cognitive reasoning abilities. An included advantage is that exercise also reduces stress and even anxiety.

The majority of doctors recommend a minimum of 30 minutes of moderate-intensity workout on a lot of days in a week.

HOW REGULAR EXERCISE CAN HELP YOUR CHILD'S BEHAVIOR

You might have currently heard that regular exercise can give your state of mind an increase. If you have ADHD, an exercise does more than make you feel great. It can help regulate your symptoms, also.

Even a single session of moving your body can make you more inspired for mental tasks, raise your psychic ability, give you energy, and also help you feel less confused. It acts upon your brain in a lot of similarities as your ADHD medication.

To reap these benefits, however, you require to exercise the proper way as well as the correct amount. The trick is to discover an activity that fits your lifestyle and then persevere.

Get the Most out of Moving Around

The results of exercise last for so long, much like medicine. Consider your workout as a therapy "dose." Go for at the very least one 30- to 40-minute task a day, 4 or 5 days a week.

The exercise you choose depends on you, but make sure it's "reasonably extreme," which means that during your workout:

Your heart rate rises

You take a breath more challenging and also quicker

You sweat

Your muscular tissues feel exhausted

Talk to your doctor if you're unclear how intense your exercise should be. She may recommend you utilize a heart rate screen or some other tool to make sure you obtain one of the most out of your workout.

Kinds of Exercise You Can Do

Aerobic exercise. Itis anything that gets your heart pounding. You wish to do something that elevates your heart rate and also maintains it there for a set quantity of time, like half an hr to 40 mins.

Cardiovascular exercise develops new pathways in your mind as well as floods it with the chemicals that help you listen.

You can attempt among these:

Running

Strolling quickly

Cycling

Swimming laps

You can do these tasks outdoors or inside, but if you have an option, go outside. Researches show that remaining in nature while you relocate can reduce your ADHD signs and symptoms a lot more than when you exercise within.

Martial arts. Experts say the extra complex your exercise is, the far better for your mind. Sports like martial arts, taekwondo, jiujitsu, as well as judo focus on self-discipline as well as bringing together your mind and body. When you do martial arts, you obtain training in abilities like:

Focus and focus

Equilibrium

Timing

Memory

Effects of activities

Fine electric motor abilities

Other complex exercises. If fighting styles aren't your thing, other physical activities that also challenge your mind and body are:

Rock climbing up

Dance

Gymnastics

Yoga

Strength training. If you're only just starting with exercise, go for cardio activities like strolling or jogging at. After you've gone to it for some time, add in some stamina work for range. Attempt workouts like:

Lunges

Squats

Pushups

Pullups

Weight training

Team sporting activities. If you join a softball or football organization, it may be merely the thing to obtain you up and also moving several times a week. Organized sports have all the benefits of exercise with the added benefit of a social team to motivate you.

Team effort refines your communication skills as well as aids you analyze your activities and also strategy in advance. Being part of a group can additionally enhance your self-worth.

How to Keep at It

Much like medication, exercise helps you treat ADHD if you keep it up. If you have issues with the focus span, how do you remain the course?

Try these ideas:

Maintain it intriguing. Switch over the kind of exercise. You can stay out of a rut if you alter your activity daily or weekly.

Locate a partner. An exercise buddy can help you stay on track as well as help kill time while you sweat.

Move-in the morning. If it fits in your routine, exercise first thing in the early morning before you take your medication. That way, you'll get the most gain from all the extra mood-boosting chemicals in your body.

Maintain meds. Exercise can give you a substantial upper hand on your ADHD signs. However, it does not change your medication. Do not stop your other therapies unless your doctor claims it's ALRIGHT.

How To Help Kids Manage ADHD With Yoga

Attention Deficit Disorder (ADHD) is a condition that appears in early childhood, with signs and symptoms that generally appear before the age of seven.

If your youngster has ADHD or you collaborate with youngsters with ADHD, you might take into consideration trying different therapies like yoga. Yoga has been shown in research studies to be an appealing treatment for kids with ADHD.

You can do yoga exercises at home with children with ADHD or obtain a professional yoga direction. You should after that, create a yoga exercise routine so the youngster can reap the benefits of this technique.

Educate your child to identify sensations in their body. Various feelings and also degrees of power will be felt differently by your child. They may feel like they have butterflies in their belly or are buzzing with electricity at times when they're hyper. Conversely, they may feel lighter sometimes when they're loosened up. Finding out to see these sensations will help them see exactly how yoga exercise affects them.

Ask your kid to rank their energy degree on a scale of 1 to 10 before and after yoga. It will undoubtedly help them see the advantages.

Make yoga enjoyable for your kid.

Attach the yoga to something that your child delights in to ensure that they'll be much more open up to trying it. For instance, you might call it "superhero training" to interest a kid that likes superhero. You might even relabel the presents to make them sound more enjoyable to your child.

Teach your kids to enjoy their breath.

Being aware of their breath will undoubtedly help your youngster experience the full benefits of yoga. Initially, instruct your kid to monitor their breathing. Once they obtain utilized to that, you can guide them just how to breathe in and exhale with each present.

Show them how to extend their breath by gradually inhaling.

Describe just how they can strengthen their breaths by pulling the air right into their tummy as well as lungs. Inform them that it takes technique, so they should do their best.

Concentrate on movement-based yoga.

After you show your kid to check their breath, show them just how to relocate via the poses. Ask your youngster to imitate an animal, transferring through poses like feline pose, downward dog, roaring lion position, and cobra present. Urge them to relocate slow activity, watching their breath.

Doing Yoga In Your Home

Beginning with Mountain Pose.

Hill's present is a great introductory present that you can do with youngsters with ADHD. Establish a yoga mat in an open space in your home and also open the yoga session with Mountain position to help the child concentrate on the practice.

To reveal the child exactly how to do Mountain Pose, stand straight with your feet with each other. Increase and also spread your toes so they are level on the mat. Straighten your legs without securing at the knees.

Ground down by pressing through your big toes and also raise your head, keeping your face onward and even your head degree. Place your hands by your sides with your hands available to the front of the room.

Hold Mountain position for ten deep inhales and breathes out. You might have the youngster matter the breaths with you to keep them focused.

Practice Roaring Lion Pose.

Roaring Lion position is a simple yoga exercise present that can help your youngster relax and also have a good time on the mat. The concept is to roar like a lion in the jungle in this present, making the most vicious face you can summon.

To do this posture with the child, kneel on the yoga exercise mat with your bottom hand on your calves. Position your hands on your knees and stay upright.

Open your mouth as well as close your eyes. Prolong your tongue out as well as down, wrinkling your nose. Inhale and afterwards as you breathe out, release a "ROARRRR" sound.

Repeat this audio five times for five breaths in total. It can be fun to do this position before a mirror, as you reach holler at your very own representation.

Do Tree Pose.

Tree pose benefits focus and concentration. It is likewise an excellent challenge for kids with ADHD to stay concentrated enough to maintain their balance.

Begin by standing with your palms along with your thumbs at your breast bone. Maintain your hands together and also slowly increase your hands over your head. Lower them back down to the beginning placement. Repeat this several times, integrating your breathing with an upward movement and also your respiration with a descending motion.

Add on the harmonizing element by focusing on an unmoving spot on the floor 4 feet far from you. Increase your appropriate leg and also location your best foot against your left calf, with your bent leg facing the ideal side.

Hold this pose for five breaths and afterwards launch. Switch over to the other side, lifting your left foot as well as placing it versus your right calf.

Practice Superman Pose.

This posture can help the kid come to be a lot more aware of their body language as well as feel more grounded. They might also enjoy the experience of "flying" on the ground.

To do Superman Pose, relax on your belly with your arms stretched overhead and your legs straight behind you. Start by inhaling as well as raising your arms off the ground. Exhale and also place your arms back on the ground. Do the very same with your legs, lifting and lowering your legs with your take a breath.

As soon as the youngster appears comfortable with training and also decreasing their arm or legs, you can attempt the complete posture. Inhale as well as lift both your limbs off the ground. You need to seem like you're flying like a superhero. Breathe out and also reduce your arm or legs. Repeat this pose for 4 to 5 complete breaths.

Attempt Drawbridge Pose.

This pose is good for focusing the youngster as well as permitting them to have even more control over the motion of their body. It is an excellent present to likewise help your youngster unwind, especially if they seem to be getting flustered or active.

Begin by pushing your back with your arms at hand, and your palms deal with down. Bend your knees and also put your feet flat on the ground. They must be hip-width apart and close sufficient that you can touch your heels with your hands.

Inhale as you press firmly right into your feet and also hands. Lift your hips off the ground like the raising of a drawbridge. After that, breathe out as you lower your hips down to the floor.

Repeat this pose for four to 5 breaths. As soon as you are done, hug your knees to your chest for 5 to ten breaths.

Relax with Child's Pose.

This pose is fantastic for concluding a yoga session or as a last yoga posture before bed. You can show the kid to enter into this pose if they start to feel overloaded or hyper, as it can be extremely relaxing as well as relaxing.

To do Child's Pose, stoop down and sit on your feet with your knees divided. You might allow your knees to develop a broad "v" form on the floor covering. Inhale and put your forehead on the ground before your knees, curving your back. Prolong your arms ahead and also take a breath genuinely in this pose for 2 to 5 minutes.

Appear of the present gradually, lifting your arms and also head. Relax on your feet as well as take a few cleaning breaths to finish your practice.

Obtaining Professional Yoga Instruction

Seek a yoga exercise course for kids with ADHD in your area.

Not all yoga exercise educators will undoubtedly be experienced sufficient to deal with kids with ADHD. You need to search for a yoga exercise class instructed by an instructor who has a strong foundation in yoga and also is familiar with how to communicate with people with ADHD. The teacher may be accredited to deal with developmentally tested youngsters or have substantial experience mentor kids with ADHD.

The majority of yoga courses for youngsters with ADHD will have 2 to 3 youngsters at once. It will enable the yoga exercise educator to function patiently as well as very carefully with each youngster.

Watch yoga exercise videos online.

You can obtain expert yoga exercise guidelines on a budget by searching for yoga exercise videos online that focus on poses for people with ADHD. You may register for a couple of video channels on the internet so you can see brand-new video clips weekly and integrate them right into yoga exercise sessions with the youngster.

You may likewise ask parents or teachers who deal with children with ADHD for recommendations on yoga video channels or websites.

Hire a private yoga exercise teacher.

You may select hiring a yoga instructor for private lessons for the youngster, so they get one on one focus. Try to find a yoga trainer who is accredited to show youngsters with ADHD and also who has worked with children with ADHD before. The teacher needs to appear person, confident, and even open with the youngster in the one on one sessions.

The instructor might also include quick routines in their sessions, like illumination incense or setting up a floor covering, so the kid obtains utilized to concentrating on details tasks. They may then do a collection of poses, making an effort to get the child to focus as well as relax during the session.

Developing a Yoga Routine

Have a deep breathing session daily.

Starting a yoga exercise routine with the child can benefit them over time. It can likewise make them more comfy with doing yoga and also in time, get even more self-confidence. You may start by setting aside time in the youngster's schedule to do deep breathing once daily. In-depth breathing sessions can be an excellent way to help your kid focus and unwind. They can after that make use of a deep breath when they are doing yoga poses.

You can sit with the child in a peaceful, darkened space in a comfortable position to do deep breathing. Try to do at the very least 10 to fifteen slow deep inhales as well as exhales. You might have the youngster location one hand on their belly and also one hand on their chest to help them get utilized to breathing in and breathing out deeply.

Do a couple of yoga exercises presents before bed.

You may also urge the kid to do a couple of relaxing yoga poses before they go to bed. You may do them together as a component of the youngster's going to bed routine. Doing unwinding positions before bed can help the kid settle down and also get in rest mode.

Make this enjoyable for your child! You could show them to do a couple of postures before bed to "trigger sleep mode," after that, a few presents in the morning to "trigger wake setting."

You might do Mountain Pose, Drawbridge Pose, and also Child's Pose together before bed. Make sure you synchronize your activities with your inhales and breathes out.

Set up the standard once a week yoga session.

You need to attempt to have once week yoga sessions with the kid so they obtain used to doing the yoga exercise positions as well as more positive doing them. You might register the kid in a regular yoga exercise course for kids with ADHD or schedule an exclusive yoga exercise session.

You may also have your very own sessions at home with the child, so they obtain utilized to doing yoga at the very least when a week.

Do yoga exercise outside to help the child emphasis.

If you discover the kid is having difficulties focusing on the yoga exercise presents, you may attempt moving the session exterior. Studies have shown that children with ADHD have far better focus when they are outdoors in natural, environment-friendly atmospheres.

You might move the yoga exercise sessions to your yard or an eco-friendly space by your home. You might likewise attempt to have a few of the yoga sessions inside as well as some sessions outdoors so the youngster feels they have variety.

Differ, the yoga presents you make with the kid.

Youngsters with ADHD succeed with energetic, differed knowing. They tend to get tired quickly and come to be distracted as soon as they have lost interest in a task. You can keep the kid concentrated by doing various yoga postures or the same yoga poses in various order during the yoga exercise sessions.

You may also attempt to include other exercises with yoga, so the child feels tested and boosted.

If you take the child to a yoga exercise class, make sure the trainer differs the yoga poses performed in the class week to week so the youngster remains engaged.

Encourage your youngster to find up with their positions.

WHY A SIMPLE CHANGE IN ATTITUDE MAY WORK WONDERS

As a parent, you certainly enjoy your youngsters quite. However, you may become annoyed when they misbehave. Kids will undoubtedly act out as a method to seek attention, press limits, or to mimic the habits of others. On top of that, youngsters require advice creating their coping skills to handle their emotions; when that is lacking, your youngsters might act out. Your kid may act out in troublesome times or in devastating means, which can be tiring. Taking steps in the direction of changing and also enhancing your youngsters' poor habits will be beneficial for your children in both the brief as well as long-term, while likewise making your life simpler.

Connect Your Expectations For Your Child's Behavior.

Youngsters require to understand what you expect from them. Rest your youngster down in a peaceful location and also clarify to him/her what sort of behaviors you intend to see, using clear information. Concentrate on correcting one habit each time. Giving your youngster a lengthy listing of items for renovation can be frustrating.

Tell him/her points like, "When you are at school, you need to listen to your educator," or you could state, "I do not desire you to strike other youngsters, also if they are implied to you."

Set Realistic Expectations

Set high assumptions for your kids, but not so high they are unreachable. You want your youngsters to have to function as well as think of what you expect. However, they must likewise be able to achieve what you are asking from them. Or else, they may seem like failings and also deal with minimized self-confidence. You also need to make sure that your assumptions are age-appropriate.

Establish an expectation like "I expect you to turn up to course promptly as well as be considerate to your teachers," rather than "I anticipate you to be a straight-A student."

Anticipating your 4-year-old never ever to lose his/her mood is unrealistic. However, expecting him/her to control his/her temper and not hit other youngsters is sensible.

Follow your very own regulations.

Youngsters see what you do and will undoubtedly tend to duplicate your actions as well as actions. If they see you disregarding to follow an expectation you made, they will undoubtedly presume they can ignore it.

Bear in mind that youngsters usually find out by example. For that reason, if you shout instead of going over things with them, then they will most likely embrace these actions. Or, if you do disappoint regard for authority numbers, then your children may likewise demonstrate comparable disrespect for their teachers, trains, moms and dads of their pals, and even you.

Keep your expectations consistent for each scenario.

Remain active and do not transform the assumption for each different circumstance. Hold your youngsters to the very same standard, whether they are going to institution, church, or the supermarket. Refer back to your composed checklist of assumptions before every new occasion to guarantee both you and your youngster recognize what is expected.

For example, if you have set a "no outbursts" plan, do not give in if your child throws a temper tantrum in the supermarket. Follow up with whatever effects you have set. If you change your assumption to get your child to stop the negative actions, he/she will undoubtedly find out that he/she can push your limitations by misbehaving.

Consistency constructs trust funds between you as well as your youngster. It will assist frame you as dependable, and also reinforce the bond in between both of you.

Uniformity will also help reduce the "presuming" your youngster may feel regarding how to behave in specific scenarios, making them a lot more protected as well as most likely to act much better.

Do not negotiate your assumptions with your youngsters.

You are the parent, so you have to set as well as adhere to the regulations you make. If your child suggests with you, advise him/her that what is anticipated of him/her has been set out, as well as he/she is responsible for promoting what you have discussed.

If you have established the assumption that your child has to finish his/her research before he/she can play his/her video clip game, you need not let him attempt to negotiate his/her way out of doing his/her homework.

If you provide into discussing with your kids, you immediately stop corresponding. If your youngsters realize they can negotiate with you about what is anticipated of them, they will not take you or the behavioral assumptions seriously.

Nevertheless, it's additionally essential to take notice of the scenario. If your boy is arguing regarding not cleaning his/her teeth, ask him/her why he/she doesn't desire to. You could learn that he has a loose tooth that injures when he/she brushes it. Lots of youngsters say when they don't recognize how else to share their sensations, especially sensations of discomfort or frustration.

Maintain in mind that arrangement can be a positive thing when your children get older. It can boost communication between you and your teen as well as make it much easier to understand each other. Allowing your teenager to negotiate with, you can also advertise vital thinking and even diplomacy. Also, it does not mean that you have to give up, just that you need to agree to pay attention.

Transforming Bad Behavior

Be proactive! Stopping poor actions before it also begins is essential.

Find out the patterns of your kid's actions so you can be prepared to do something about it. If you recognize your youngster is going to call for your focus throughout an essential phone call, involve her in a challenge or a TELEVISION show that will hold her interest for the duration of your telephone call.

Be clear with your youngster, informing her specifically what is going to take place. Before your phone call, state something like, "Mommy will certainly be on the phone for 10 mins. I require you not to disrupt me. I have put in your Ice Age DVD and have some yummy apples for you. When I am done on the phone, I will certainly come to cuddle as well as a treat with you!"

If you understand that your youngster often tends to act out when he/she is tired or hungry, make sure that he/she has enough treats and gets a great night's rest.

Pay attention to your child.

Excellent communication is the most critical tool in your parenting toolbox. When your youngster misbehaves, put in the time to ask your youngster what took place, as well as listen to her when he/she describes.

Say your son/daughter has struck his/her good friend. Ask him/her about what happened. You might uncover that he/she hit his/her friend because the close friend would not share a plaything, or because he/she is starving or tired and unable to express those feelings suitably.

Restate what your kid has informed you. It is an energetic listening technique, as well as modeling it for your children, which will undoubtedly assist create their communication skills. For instance, you could say, "I'm hearing you state that you felt mad that your friend would not share. Is that right?"

Speak to your children concerning their feelings.

As soon as you have listened, seize the day to mention areas for development in your kid's actions.

You could tell your son/daughter, "You were feeling upset since your buddy wouldn't share. It isn't enjoyable to feel dismayed, is it?" When he/she agrees, you can adhere to up with "When you hit your close friend, it made him/her feel distressed, as well. Do you believe he/she likes feeling disturbed?" This sort of dialogue will encourage your kid to consider how others feel and the consequences of her actions.

Make a plan for the following time your child feels this way.

It's essential to assist your children in making a plan for what to do when they experience feelings that disturb them and also could result in acting out. This type of action plan is typically utilized for kids with ADHD, but it's an excellent idea for all kids. You and your son/daughter might come up with a plan that consists of the following steps for the next time he/she feels upset:

Take a few deep breaths.

Spend time in another room to cool down.

Describe what made him/her trouble.

Work out the remedy to his/her issue with moms and dad or in between his/her brother or sister or good friends.

Discuss why you have guidelines.

Frequently, children will act out because they don't understand why they are meant to comply with the policies and expectations you have established. Clarify to your youngster specifically why he/she has to adhere to the system you have established him/her.

For instance, if your son/daughter tosses his/her toys about, you could tell him/her: "We have a guideline that you can't toss your playthings. Throwing your toys could damage them or hurt somebody. It's unsafe, which's why you are not allowed to do it."

Attempt advising your child concerning the "why" the very first time or two he/she breaks the policy. For instance, if you see your son/daughter throwing his/her plaything, ask him/her, "Why do we have the regulation about not tossing playthings?" It will motivate him/her to keep in mind why he/she is not allowed to throw toys.

Follow through and do not give vacant guarantees.

Following up with your words and satisfying your assurances starts to establish count on as well as regard for you as a parent. If you tell your child you will certainly cuddle with him/her, make sure to do so. Otherwise, your child will not trust you and will be more likely to act out and also "call your bluff."

Children are smart as well as will certainly remember what you say. They will certainly likewise attempt to press the limits. You have to remain true to your sentences as well as established limitations for your children.

You likewise have to follow through when you are correcting negative behaviors. If you inform your child that you will undoubtedly remove his/her playthings if he remains to toss them, after that, be sure to take them away if the proceeds of the imperfect action, regardless of your child's unavoidable protests.

Encourage your kids by providing options.

Attempt offering the power to your kid by giving him/her options in a circumstance. Be strategic in the choices you supply him/her by making both alternatives appropriate habits. For example, claim something like, "You can either get dressed for school now or eat breakfast first." In either case, they are doing what you want in a way you consider acceptable.

Attempt offering your children severe choices that give them no selection but to act. "You can pick to remain here with your good friend yet share and also be good, or you can choose to leave." By doing this, the child is compelled to behave well if he/she intends to remain to have fun.

Show favorable actions instead of negative ones to get the same result.

Your kid is likely tossing toys while you get on a phone call to obtain focus. If you educate your kid to ask well instead and wait patiently for attention, he will undoubtedly achieve the same result while acting suitably.

If you are asking your kid to wait a few more minutes before he/she will certainly get interest, try making use of a timer to give both of you a concrete concept of the length of time till the kid gets what you guaranteed.

Award Good Behavior.

Children look for and also require attention, and will undoubtedly seek it in both positive as well as negative ways. Providing positive support aids your child to learn what they are doing well, and makes them intend to duplicate that etiquette.

Be very confident in your applauds, by stating things like "Great job cleansing your area as I asked. Thank you!" or "That was fantastic how you shared your toys with your close friends." Or, you can additionally attempt subtle favorable support with smiles, responds, and also hugs.

Producing Effective Consequences

Set out the effects of harmful habits up-front.

When you describe your assumptions permanently behavior, additionally explains the consequences for disobeying the expectation. By doing this, your youngster can choose precisely how to act while understanding accurately what will happen. Say something like, "I anticipate you to hold my hand when we cross the street, and if you do not, you will have to spend ten minutes in time-out." It will create your child to believe even more deeply before he/she takes part in harmful behaviors.

Make each repercussion short as well as easy to understand to raise the chance of your child remembering them. For example, "No iPad today," "No Sesame Street today," or "30 minutes deducted from your computer time today."

Discuss why your child is receiving an effect.

When you implement a repercussion, make sure your child recognizes why he/she is being penalized. Plainly describe to him/her that you have talked about with him/her what is anticipated, he/she disobeyed you, so now he/she needs to deal with the repercussion. By clearly discussing the effects, there is no area for complications concerning what behavior was wrong, as well as you will both be on the same web page.

Attempt stating something like, "We both concurred that you would certainly not hit other kids when they do not share their playthings. Because you hit your close friend, you will certainly not get to play your computer game tonight."

Deal A Choice Of Tangible Rewards When Your Child Engages In Desired Behavior.

Favorable reinforcement is the most positive consequence. When your kid behaves in a way that you approve, use him/her an item of candy, and added 10 mins on the playground, or a sticker label.

You can attempt "huge" rewards if your child is exceptionally well behaved for an extensive amount of time such as having a sleepover, obtaining ice cream, or choosing one thing from the toy store.

Reward, yet do not reward! Rewarding occurs after a behavior is a total, while allurements arise before the truth. If you are approaching your kid to act well, he/she may come to be baffled and also think he/she needs to function well when he/she makes money.

Ensure your benefit suits the habits. Using a sticker for sitting through the church silently is acceptable. Yet offering a sticker label for not hitting a classmate could not be a grand adequate incentive. Adapt and adapt to each situation.

Make repercussions short of optimizing their performance.

Kids can typically be absent-minded as well as a result, if you make a specific effect last also long, they may fail to remember why they are being punished. If you take your child's toys away since he/she was throwing them, do so just for a few hours or a day, not for a week or a month.

Furthermore, long-term consequences might bring about increased negative habits. For instance, if you ground your kid for two months, he might think, "Why should I act? I'm currently based".

Always attempt talking to your youngster first to find out what is going on. Punishment should be used as a last option.

Be consistent.

Picking to institute effects when it is hassle-free for you is confusing as well as undermines your authority as a parent. By not corresponding, your kid may likewise become puzzled regarding when poor actions will undoubtedly be faced with an effect, and also this will likely cause aggravated behaviors.

HOW TO DISCOVER THE VERY BEST THERAPY FOR YOUR KID

Behavior modification is a reliable therapy for attention-deficit/hyperactivity disorder (ADHD) that can improve a youngster's habits, self-control, and self-confidence. It is most truthful in kids when moms and dads supply it. Specialists recommend that doctors refer moms and dads of kids more youthful than 12 years of age for training in behavior therapy. For kids younger than six years of age, parent training in behavior monitoring should be attempted before prescribing ADHD medicine.

When moms and dads become learned behavior modification, they find out skills as well as methods to assist their kid with ADHD to do well at college, in your home, and also in connections. Understanding and practicing behavior therapy requires time and effort. However, it has enduring advantages for the youngster and the family members.

Did you know?

Parent training in habits administration is likewise called moms and dad behavior therapy, behavioral moms and dad training, or only parent training.

What should parents seek?

Preferably, family members ought to look for a specialist who focuses on training parents. Some specialists will have training or accreditation in moms and dad training program that has been confirmed to work in young children with ADHD.

Therapists may likewise utilize techniques like those in proven programs1,2. The adhering to a listing of concerns can be used to find a specialist that utilizes a proven method:

Does this therapist

Teach moms and dads skills as well as techniques that use favorable support, framework, as well as a convenient routine to manage their kid's habits?

Show parents favorable methods to communicate and interact with their kids?

Appoint activities for parents to exercise with their kids?

Meet regularly with the family to monitor development and also supply mentoring and support?

Re-evaluate therapy plans, as well as stay adaptable adequate to change strategies as needed?

Learn more about finding a specialist "

What can parents expect?

Parents usually participate in 8 or even more sessions with a therapist. Sessions might involve dealing with groups of moms and dads or with one family member alone. The therapist meets regularly with the moms and dads to assess their development, offer assistance, and readjust strategies, as required, to make sure renovation. Parents typically practice with their child between sessions.

Parents have the best impact on their kid's behavior. Just treatment that focuses on training moms and dads is suggested for kids with ADHD because children are not fully grown enough to transform their habits without their parents' aid. Some therapists might make use of play therapy or talk therapy to treat kids with ADHD. Play treatment offers a way for children to communicate their experiences and also sensations through play. Talk therapy utilizes verbal communication in between the kid and even a specialist to treat mental and mental illness. Neither of these has been shown to enhance symptoms in children with ADHD.

Learning and also practicing behavior modification requires time and effort, but it has long-lasting advantages for the youngster. Ask your doctor concerning the benefits of moms and dad training in behavior modification for young kids with ADHD.

What can healthcare providers do?

Doctor can:

Follow the scientific practice standard for medical diagnosis and therapy of ADHD in young children an external symbol

Review with parents the benefits of behavior therapy as well as why they ought to take into consideration getting training.

Recognize parent training service providers in their location and also refer moms and dads of young children with ADHD for training in behavior modification before suggesting medicine.

TREATING YOUR CHILD'S ADHD

Observe difficulties with focus. There two kinds of ADHD signs. For kids under 17, a minimum of 6 of these must exist for an ADHD diagnosis. For older individuals, only five are needed — the first collection of signs associated with issues with focus or emphasis.

They include:

Making negligent errors, being unobserving to information

Having a problem focusing (tasks, playing).

They are not seeming to listen when a person is talking.

Not following up on research, chores, or work, conveniently averted.

It is being organizationally tested.

Avoiding jobs needing continual focus.

Not tracking or commonly losing products such as tricks, glasses, and so on

. Being conveniently sidetracked.

Frequently forgetting things.

Hyperactivity.

The various other group ADHD symptoms associated with hyperactivity or absence of impulse control.

Expect the following:

Fidgeting or agonizing; tapping hands or feet.

Feeling troubled, running, or climbing up inappropriately.

Having a hard time to remain quiet.

Speaking exceedingly.

They are spouting out answers before inquiries are asked.

Having a hard time to await his/her turn.

Disturbing others.

Discover the causes of ADHD.

The brain of an individual with ADHD is somewhat various than others. Two frameworks specifically tend to be smaller sized: the basal ganglia and the prefrontal cortex.

The first ganglia regulate the motion of muscular tissues.

It indicates which must be working as well as which must be at rest at any offered time.

If a kid is resting at a work desk in the classroom, the first ganglia needs to send out a message informing the feet to remain still. In the case of ADHD, the feet may not obtain the news. They may stay in motion. A shortage of the basic ganglia can likewise often cause fidgety hand motions. For example, individuals with ADHD might touch a pencil on a desk or drum their fingers.

The prefrontal cortex is essential for conducting higher-order jobs.

It is where memory, discovering, and focus law come together. This area is necessary for intellectual features.

The prefrontal cortex plays an essential function in managing natural chemical dopamine.

Dopamine influences your ability to focus and usually is at reduced degrees face to faces with ADHD.

Serotonin is one more neurotransmitter related to the prefrontal cortex. It affects mood, rest, and also appetite. When serotonin drops as well reduced, clinical depression as well as stress and anxiety result.

Lower degrees of dopamine and serotonin can make it harder to focus. Because of this, individuals with

ADHD struggle to concentrate on one thing at a time and are more easily sidetracked.

Look out for relevant problems.

ADHD commonly occurs together with various other mental health issues. It is called "comorbidity.".

One in 5 individuals with ADHD likewise has some other significant disorder. Depression and bipolar affective disorder are the most common.

One in 3 youngsters with ADHD also has a behavior condition. These include conduct problems as well as different defiance conditions.

Learning disabilities and also anxiousness likewise generally appear along with ADHD.

See a medical professional for medical diagnosis.

If you or a loved one has many of these traits, you need to see a doctor obtain an expert point of view. Understanding if ADHD might be the reason for these troubles will certainly help you pick the best therapy.

Dealing with ADHD

Obtain a prescription for the right drug.

For most individuals with ADHD, medication is a fundamental part of therapy. There are two classifications of ADHD medication: stimulants (such as methylphenidate as well as amphetamine) and also non-stimulants (such as guanfacine as well as atomoxetine).

Using stimulants to treat ADHD may not seem like it makes much feeling.

The components of the mind they stimulate, however, are accountable for impulse control and also emphasis. Energizers like Ritalin, Concerta, and also Adderall can assist in regulating neurotransmitters like norepinephrine and also dopamine.

Non-stimulant anti-depression drugs frequently used to treat ADHD manage the same neurotransmitters. They do so through a different chemical procedure. Doctors might recommend them if stimulants don't work or have rough side-effects.

Choosing the best medication can be tough.

Different individuals respond in different ways to different medications. The performance of some medicines can also transform throughout development surges, hormone fluctuations, diet plan as well as weight modifications, and with the flow of time. The best method to choose the ideal medicine is through discussion with your doctor. Bear in mind that if something does not seem to be functioning, you can speak to your medical professional concerning attempting a different choice.

Some medicines are available in extended-release varieties. They launch active ingredients progressively over the day. It removes the demand to take extra dosages at school or job.

Eat a diet regimen that combats ADHD.

Some foods can lower the effects of the hormonal shortages that are usually component of ADHD. Here are some suggestions.

Complex carbohydrates can raise serotonin degrees. It can suggest a better mood, sleep, and also appetite. Attempt to consume foods like entire grains, eco-friendly vegetables, starchy vegetables, and even beans. These foods release power progressively. Prevent necessary carbs like sugars, honey, jelly, candy, soft drink, and so on. These can create a temporary serotonin spike, yet do more injury than great over the future.

A diet plan abundant in healthy protein can boost emphasis. Try to include numerous healthy proteins throughout the day to keep dopamine degrees high. Great sources of protein consist of meat, fish, nuts, legumes, and beans.

Take zinc. Zinc advertises lower degrees of attention deficit disorder as well as impulsivity. Consume seafood, fowl strengthened grains as well as various other foods with a high zinc web content, and take zinc supplements.

Eating specific spices might also assist. Saffron may counter clinical depression, while cinnamon can aid with interest and also focus. [

Stay clear of foods that worsen ADHD.

Various other foods can sometimes make the problem worse. :.

Stay clear of "negative fats" such as trans fats and those discovered in fried foods, burgers, and pizza. Select foods high in omega-3 fatty acids rather. Excellent sources include salmon, walnuts, as well as avocados. These might assist reduced hyperactivity as well as enhance business skills.

Prevent food with dyes and also food coloring. Some studies suggest there may be a web link between food dyes and ADHD signs and symptoms. The red color in particular might be a problem.

Minimize consumption of wheat as well as dairy products, sugar, refined foods, and additives. These foods might bad ADHD signs.

Obtain treatment for ADHD.

A good therapist can help you and your loved ones handle the challenges of ADHD. Treatment usually starts by analyzing the family members' structure. The therapist will certainly typically recommend changes to create an environment that deals with the mind functions of a person with ADHD.

Treatment also offers a refuge for family members to vent their irritations in a healthy and balanced means. It is a venue to work out concerns with specialist support.

Experts commonly recommend that young children with ADHD obtain behavioral therapy. This approach educates people on exactly how to change behavior and control impulses.

Grownups with ADHD usually take advantage of psychotherapy. It aids them to accept who they are while looking for renovations to their circumstances.

Individuals with ADHD advantage significantly from discovering more about their problems. Therapy aids them to comprehend that they are not alone in their struggles.

Get plenty of exercise.

Exercise stimulates the production of much of the same neurotransmitters as ADHD medication. Extreme workouts are a fantastic way to manage your brain chemistry, but also a couple of 30 min strolls every week can make a huge difference.

Specifically, exercise promotes the production of dopamine, norepinephrine, and also serotonin. All these can assist boost focus and emphasis.

Utilizing Everyday Strategies For Coping.

Arrange the environment.

People with ADHD are continually trying to understand their settings. Organizing the residence is a fantastic method to begin.

People with ADHD frequently have difficulty bearing in mind where they put things. Having assigned containers, tubs, shelves, or hooks for different sorts of products can make life much more comfortable.

It is especially essential for children, that gain from well-arranged bedrooms and also play locations.

Assist kids to remain arranged by supplying color-coded containers as well as bathtubs. You can also identify these with photos or words explaining the types of items that belong within.

Similar business strategies can additionally benefit adults in the workplace.

Decrease distractions.

People with ADHD additionally have trouble straining disturbances in the environment. Below are a few pointers for lowering interruptions in the home or office.

Switch off the TELEVISION and stereo when you are not watching or listening. Both of these can be distracting. It is especially important when an individual with ADHD is trying to concentrate or when you are attempting to interact with children.

Readjust lights. Lighting that creates shadows or unique patterns can be distracting for individuals with ADHD. Make lights in your home regularly, and change flickering light bulbs right away. Stay away from fluorescent illumination, as the hum of the bulbs can likewise make it challenging to focus.

Avoid strong scents. Distinctive smells can likewise make it hard for someone with ADHD to focus. Prevent aromatic air fresheners, as well as fragrances as well as colognes.

Establish a routine.

People with ADHD succeed with constant routines. Doing the very same thing at the very same time and also in the exact same place each day makes it easier to bear in mind and also concentrate on essential jobs.

For youngsters, having a particular time allotted for homework and also tasks is helpful. It can additionally reduce disagreements around these topics.

Breaking routine tasks down into small, convenient pieces likewise assists. Individuals with ADHD have a problem holding great deals of instructions in their heads at the very same time. Even things that appear simple can be simplified. Filling the dishwasher can be damaged up into packing the top rack, lower shelf, and silverware.

For young people with ADHD, appreciation and also little incentives at each action can aid enhance the pattern. For deviations, instant, as well as a regular discipline, can additionally help. Make sure the effects of wrongdoing coincide every time and also come swiftly after the actions.

Developing a framework throughout school breaks is specifically crucial for children and teenagers. Urge them to sign up with assigned tasks that have standard conferences. Examples include summertime supply plays, sports groups, or clubs.

Utilize a planner.

Keeping a planner or schedule can be useful for people with ADHD. It can be a place to tape-record the everyday routine, along with details jobs like homework or job conferences.

A coordinator is most handy if you inspect and upgrade it often.

You can use applications or on-line planners with visible or audible suggestions to make sure you do not forget visits or set up jobs.

For kids, it is a great idea to ask teachers to be preliminary the planner every day to make sure the pupil has taped homework correctly.

Looking For Help in School or the Workplace.

Obtain assistance in school. Schools supply numerous services for kids with ADHD.

These services range from extra time on tests to self-supporting classes with specially trained teachers and aides.

Interact with educators to make sure they understand the nature of the child's condition. Some educators error ADHD for stubbornness or an attitude problem.

Ask for individual education evaluation. It will allow you to work with the school to produce an Individual Education Plan (IEP) for the student. This document specifies goals for the pupil, along with interventions and also strategies for getting to those goals. Make sure to send the assessment request in creating.

You'll produce an IEP busy with school officials. Do not permit the school to pressure you right into signing a "one-size-fits-all" IEP. It needs to be customized to the needs of the individual student.

Get a help-seeking job.

There are additionally might service offered for people with ADHD that are looking for employment. These are provided by colleges, state companies, and also non-profit organizations.

A variety of transitional solutions are readily available to aid school-aged youngsters to apply for college, professional school, or jobs. It includes help with filling out applications, talking to, and also independent living. Transitional solutions must be the focus of IEPs for pupils over the age of 16.

All states in the US deal with employment rehab (VR) services. These are services for individuals with disabilities who need aid looking for or keeping work. Virtual Reality therapists can sometimes help with financial help to a university or vocational training camp. For instance, a VR program could sponsor truck-driving classes to obtain an industrial driver's permit. Search your state federal government's website to see what solutions are available.

Other Virtual Reality services may include the computer of job abilities training. A Virtual Reality program may supply hearing aids or various other flexible modern technology. It may also provide help completing applications or producing resumes, and practicing interviewing abilities.

Obtain help in maintaining work. People with ADHD often battle to keep tasks.

Issues with emphasis, time administration, and also, in some cases, social abilities create obstacles to rewarding work. Here are a few suggestions for obtaining help.

Connect with managers and coworkers concerning the limitations that feature ADHD. If they find out about the problem, they are most likely to be thoughtful as well as consider it.

Virtual Reality solutions additionally offer training that can make it simpler to function at the office. They can help with work abilities as well as the organization. Again, examine the state's internet site to see what solutions are readily available.

You can employ a task coach that will undoubtedly go through your workday with you. He or she will search for issues as well as make recommendations to you and also your employer for making your work extra efficient and even productive. Virtual Reality solutions typically offer or spend on task mentoring. Charitable organizations in your area might likewise provide this service.

RESOURCES FOR PARENTS AS WELL AS KIDS WITH ADHD

Resources for ADHD

Attention deficit disorder (ADHD) is just one of the most typical childhood neurodevelopmental conditions. It affects as much as 5 percent Trusted Source of kids in the United States.

According to the American Psychiatric Association (APA), approximately 2.5 percent of adults likewise deal with this condition. Men are three times most likely to be diagnosed with ADHD than females.

Youngsters, as well as adults with ADHD, might deal with impulse control, hyperactivity, as well as problems paying attention for extended periods. Left neglected, it can interrupt one's capability to process, comprehend, as well as find out details.

Numerous sources and treatments-- such as medication and behavioral therapy-- can assist those with ADHD who live satisfying and useful lives. There are additionally a variety of organizations, resources, and also academic devices-- like the ones listed below-- that can aid those with ADHD and their friends and family.

Not-for-profit companies

Nonprofit companies can be a practical resource, using valuable info regarding ADHD, along with info for friends and family members.

Below are companies that supply sources for kids, as well as grownups coping with ADHD Not-for-profit organizations found in Canada as well as the United Kingdom, are also consisted of.

CHADD: The National Resource for ADHD.

Attention Deficit Disorder Association (ADDA).

Centre for ADHD Awareness, Canada (CADDAC).

ADHD Foundation: Mental Health, Education, and Training Services.

The American Professional Society of ADHD as well as Related Disorders.

ADHD World Federation: Child and Adult Disorder.

Kid Mind Institute.

SETTING ROUTINES/HABITS FOR A CHILD WITH ADHD

Kids with ADHD need routine. Trusted schedules for mornings, after school, and bedtime make an incredible distinction in establishing expectations, building desirable behaviors, as well as improving ADD-related habits. Utilize these suggested layouts to wrangle your family members' time.

All parents of children with ADHD have listened to the routine concerning routines: Kids require a framework, as well as children with attention-deficit, require a lot more. The tricks to obtaining the ADHD company aid you need: idea in the power of family regimens and also a lasting dedication to them.

You've heard it before: Set up an early morning routine for youngsters with ADHD to go out the door on schedule. Make sure research happens at the same time as well as in the very same setting daily. Do something fun to loosen up before a regular bedtime.

Theoretically, this appears pretty necessary. When you're raising a child with actual focus troubles in the genuine globe, establishing and keeping such routines can seem downright helpless. Yet there is hope-- also a joy-- insight.

Many sympathetic moms and dads enthusiastically start to establish the structure their kids require. Yet lots of surrender after a couple of weeks (or even a few days) because the regimens are not functioning. "Billy will not listen. He does not wish to accompany it. Each day comes to be a fight, and we're all worn. Is there another thing we can try?"

Usually, trying to execute a day-to-day routine doesn't function since parents give up prematurely. To make structure genuinely reliable, regimens require to be seen as well as implemented not equally as basic behavioral techniques; however, as a way of living.

The Benefits of placing Your Child on a Schedule

Regimens impact life favorably on 2 degrees. In regards to habits, they help enhance performance and day-to-day functioning. It may not always be apparent, but kids want as well as require routines. A foreseeable method offers a structure that helps kids feel safe and safe and secure. By developing one, you send out a message that states, "This is how we do things." Routines make everyday tasks convenient, allowing your child to focus on one thing at a time.

Additionally, your entire family will benefit mentally from a structured regimen. Both parents and kids experience lowered stress when there's much less dramatization regarding what time you'll eat supper and also where you'll calm down to do research.

What follows is a relaxed residence, which generates stronger family partnerships. And also, family member's identification is solidified by routines in which every person contributes (Anna sets the table, Brian clears the meals). The message: We are relatives who eat together; we are family members that read with each other; we are a family who routines standard times for schoolwork and also other ongoing responsibilities.

In these desperate times, it might appear challenging to give a structured way of life. Every person is juggling timetables: job, school, entertainment, music lessons, basketball technique, and so on. Yet in just such times, the structure ends up being crucial. The benefit: higher productivity for your youngster, in addition to better wellness and also household relationships.

A review of 50 years of psychological research study, just recently released in the Journal of Family Psychology, shows that even infants, as well as young children, are healthier and display better-regulated habits when there are predictable routines in the household.

Effective regimens take commitment as well as consistency, with all family members adults providing a united front. Regimens should be developed when youngsters are young and used continuously as they grow-- but it's never too late to begin. Above all, don't quit.

Here are suggestions and some example routines to assist obtain you began. You'll want to modify them to match the age as well as the maturation of your youngster, the specific actions you are working on, as well as your family's character as well as needs. As you establish your regimens, bear in mind that success takes some time-- often months and also years. Yet the benefits will undoubtedly last a lifetime.

Greetings Start with Your Child's Schedule

The objective of the early morning routine is to obtain every person all set and also out the door on time. Preparations made the night before, such as showering, loading bookbags, outlining clothing, setting the alarm, and creating lunch, are essential in establishing a smooth morning routine.

Since lots of children (and adults) with ADHD are very distractible and also spontaneous, prevent stimuli that are likely to get focus as well as toss the routine of the training course. :

Leave the TELEVISION off in the early morning.

Do not hop on the computer system to check your e-mails.

Neglect that brand-new magazine or directory till after school or later that night.

After School Schedule: Homework Helpers

It's frequently stated that the only constant thing about children with ADHD is their disparity. This is particularly problematic when it involves academic effort. No activity demands a more significant structure and also uniformity than homework when a youngster's capability to self-regulate is called upon. Not surprisingly, parent-child homework battles are frequent. Yet a well-known study routine (time, place, approaches) goes a lengthy method toward lowering their frequency and also strength-- otherwise eliminating them. To develop a research routine that will certainly enhance efficiency as well as boost scholastic success:

Impose a regular begin time. It will assist your kid in developing a research behavior.

Stay near to your youngster. Lots of kids with ADHD concentrate much better when a grown-up work with them or neighbors.

Take breaks. Distractibility, uneasiness, trouble maintaining concentration, and also reduced irritation tolerance-- all common of ADHD-- practically guarantee psychological fatigue and monotony. Regular time-outs, during which the youngster is permitted to move, can aid.

Have a good time afterward. Your child is most likely to use herself to research when she knows that fun activity, such as playing a game or viewing TELEVISION, will undoubtedly adhere to.

A Consistent Dinnertime Schedule

For centuries, a relative has built solid relationships around the table. In this age of the Internet as well as TELEVISION films as needed, a dinner ritual is still useful, if not essential. While most nourishments last only about 20 mins (much less time than a TELEVISION comedy), a lot of good ideas can take place in that short time. Preferably, nourishments should be real social time, with business, school, or family problems left off the table. It takes time and also jobs to prepare a household meal, and also it can be trouble getting everybody together at once. Yet, you'll discover the advantages are well worth the initiative:

Members of the family stay attached to each other's lives.

Occasions are reviewed as well as prepares to obtain made with everybody's input.

Responsibility, as well as family cohesion, are motivated by such easy work as kids establishing the table and also tidying up later on.

Great Nights Begin with a Bedtime Routine

Your objective at bedtime is to aid your youngster wind down and get to rest at a typical time. Study reveals that youngsters with routine bedtime regimens get to relax sooner and also stir up much less usually throughout the night than those without them. Several kids with ADHD battle bedtime since, rather merely, going to sleep is annoying to them. It's time for rest. However, there's still so much they can do! Routines that provide benefits as well as a pleasurable activity while motivating relaxation can aid overcome the monotony of bedtime. Some points to try:

Have a light, healthy, and balanced snack, like an apple or cheese on a rice cake.

Play a quiet, low-stakes video game, or read a publication.

Have a sweet and also individual nighttime lights-out ritual.

Try to obtain your kid right into bed at the same time each night.

No question about developing family routines takes a lot of time and effort. You may ask on your own, "Can we afford the time as well as the energy to do every one of this?" A much better concern might be, "Can we pay for not to?

ADHD Organization Help: A Sample Schedule

7:00 a.m. Tickle your child out of bed. (A little delighted energy can get her up and also moving quickly.).

7:05 a.m. Get all set: Post a listing as well as have your child stick to it.

Clean face.

Brush hair.

Get dressed. (Clothes are set out the night before.) Examine to see how your youngster is doing, but let her comply with the listing and do for herself.

7:20 a.m. Breakfast time: Offer two healthy and balanced yet enticing selections, max. You would like her to spend her time eating, not yearning over Lucky Charms.

7:45 a.m. Brush your teeth-- together. Being with her can pace things up and also ensure great hygiene.

7:55 a.m. Zip, connection, and layer up. Keeping shoes and also handwear covers by the front door saves you the hide-and-seek.

8:00 a.m. Out you go.

Test Homework schedule.

3:00 p.m. Have a cookie and also relax from school.

3:30 p.m. Settle your child at his normal homework area; make sure all devices are offered (pencils, paper, calculator, referral publications, and so on).

3:35-- 4:30 p.m. Your kid does homework; you remain around to respond to questions and monitor breaks (stretch, restroom, drink).

4:25 p.m. Check his work, as well as calmly review anything he must modify (however, don't do it for him). Offer details praise job entirely.

Test Dinner schedule.

6:00 p.m. Parents start food preparation. Arrange prep work to make sure that you can stay clear of the delay of nourishment.

6:15 p.m., children set the table. Give them specific tasks to introduce a sense of obligation.

6:30 p.m. Kids put the drinks.

6:45 p.m. The mother bring the foodstuff bent on the table.

7:00 p.m. Dinner is offered. For banquet talk, try this: Go around the table-- as soon as or more-- and also have each person share one good idea concerning the child day at large

7:30 p.m. Kids clear the table. Moms and dad(s) lots the dishwasher.

Experience a Bedtime Routine.

8:00 p.m. Let him unwind in the tub. You can check out to him, or he can review it to himself. Past sanitation, a bathroom can help a child mellow out at day's end.

8:20 p.m. Three-part routine: dry off, brush teeth, as well as pee. You do not want to listen to, "Mom, I have to go to the restroom!" 5 mins after you say goodnight.

8:30 p.m. Get right into PJs and clean up toys to establish nighttime, not a play, situation.

8:40 p.m. Read together.

8:55 p.m. Your youngster gets into bed. Do your nighttime custom: Talk a little about the day, praise your child on the things he succeeded, claim your ritual goodnight-- "I like you right to the moon as well as back again. Do not let the bug bite.".

MEDICATIONS COMMONLY PRESCRIBED FOR ADHD

1. Methylphenidates: This household of energizers is utilized to treat both ADHD and narcolepsy. Trademark name are: Ritalin, Concerta, Metadate, Focalin, Daytrana

2. Dextroamphetamine: Brand names are: Exedrine, Vyvanse.

3. Amphetamines: These medications were as soon as accepted by the FDA in the 1960s for the therapy of weight problems as well as ADHD. One of the most typical brands is Adderall.

Ritalin, Concerta, Metadate, Focalin, Daytrana.

Medication bottle Ritalin, methylphenidate, is the most commonly recommended medication for ADHD. The first proposed dose is 5 mg of the short-acting range for young kids, as well as 10 mg for older youngsters, teenagers, and also grownups. The majority of people take a morning and even a lunch dosage. Some people also need a mid-afternoon dose to finish homework or various other required tasks. Clients (and caretakers) are encouraged to track action to medication and also record back to the recommending doctor. If adverse effects are marginal, the company will progressively increase the dose until the person notices enhancement. Kids, as well as their caregivers, must not boost the treatment without talking to their doctor. The maximum advised dosage of Ritalin is 60 mg per day. This higher dosage usually is tried before switching to various medications.

If Ritalin is active, and an optimum dose has been determined, the service provider may recommend switching over to long acting (LA) formula. It gets rid of the need for greater than one dosage each day. Ritalin LA is created with a 50% prompt release, as well as a 50% delayed-release. This two-tiered release prolongs the medicine's performance for approximately eight hrs. It generates two equivalent stage does, one in the morning as well as one in the mid-day. It functions well for many individuals, but not all. Locating one of the most effective dosages may call for perseverance and adaptability as various methods are checked.

Focalin is a reliable type of methylphenidate. It has only been approximately for about ten years. A productive medication activity can be beneficial in some cases for instance, some adults or enormous individuals. It may be too intense for young youngsters and may also trigger lots of side effects. Focalin can be found in a pill with 50% immediate release, and even 50% postponed the launch. It lasts for for12 hours.

Another option is Daytrana, which is a methylphenidate spot. Primarily, the place has medication that's ingrained in the adhesive. You peel the liner, and the adhesive holds it next to the skin. The drug is taken in with the skin, straight into the bloodstream. A patch offers an extra even and steady dose than pills taken in via the intestinal tract track.

Nonetheless, it takes longer to work. Once a therapeutic degree is obtained, the medication level remains very continuous for about 9 to 10 hrs or up until the spot is removed. Blood levels return to standard regarding an hr and a fifty percent after removing the patch.

Dexedrine, Exedrine,

If Ritalin does not show effective, Dexedrine, a Dextroamphetamine, is the following, probably a candidate to try. Concerning 12% of individuals with ADHD are treated with this medication. In addition to influencing dopamine levels, Dexedrine likewise affects norepinephrine degrees. Norepinephrine is an additional natural chemical that affects our capacity to pay attention as well as focus.

This medication decreases tiredness, increases electric motor task and psychological performance, and also produces moderate euphoria. The adverse effects of making use of Dexedrine consist of enhanced heart rate, blood vessel restriction, and bronchial dilation. However, the critical problem regarding its use is connected to its potential to be re-sealed as a road medicine. It is two times as powerful as Ritalin, as well as is highly valued in the underground medication trade.

A 5 mg dose lasts typically 5 to 6 hours. Using Dexedrine adds flexibility to a therapy program because there are three strengths of slow-release tablets. These are much more dependable than slow-release Ritalin; they are harder to get because they are a lot more closely monitored by the DEA.

Viviane

Vyvanse is an additional amphetamine; however, it additionally includes a substance called lysine. Lysine affixes itself to the active component in Adderall, an amphetamine. To metabolize this drug, an added action is required to disintegrate Lysine from Adderall. This combined process ensures that Vyvanse lasts a long time-up to 14 hours. Although this length of time can conveniently be also long for a little one, maybe perfect for people in senior high school or university, or a grownup. It's a powdered medication, so it will certainly have a regular launch, without peaks as well as troughs.

Adderall.

Adderall is an immediate-acting amphetamine. Its impact will certainly last for 3 to 4 hrs. Adderall XR (extended-release) is a mix of both prompt and also slow-release forms. The XR type lasts up to 10 to 12 hours (two times as lengthy as Dexedrine). The advantage of the XR kind is it generally needs only one dosage per day. Both unbiased efficiency actions (e.g., qualities, tests), as well as subjective measures (e.g., teacher scores), suggest both forms of Adderall work. The adverse effects of Adderall are similar to Dexedrine. The recommended dose for kids is 5 to 60 mg. This broad range suggests the different reactions of private kids as an outcome of dimension, metabolism, and also the age of the kid.

National Drug Administration is a company in the United States in charge of drug guidelines. In 2005, the FDA launched a warning about making use of Adderall in response to 12 pediatric deaths. With further examination, extenuating scenarios were found in each situation. These consisted of heat exhaustion, Type I diabetes, dehydration, as well as incredibly vigorous exercise. Some kids had hidden heart conditions that added to their fatality. The FDA compared the rate of premature death for these cases of pediatric Adderall individuals, versus the early death price in the general pediatric populace. This comparison revealed comparable prices.

Consequently, the FDA is remaining to explore the connection between Adderall as well as sudden death. Nonetheless, the FDA has not removed Adderall from the marketplace. Currently, there are no more limitations on Adderall, other than a warning that individuals with underlying heart disease are at particular danger.

COMPARING DRUGS FOR ADHD

	Stimulants	Non-Stimulants: Atomoxetine (Strattera) as well as Alpha-2 Adrenergics
The Way Or Manner They Work	Generally, target receptors of the brain chemical dopamine. Very efficient at	Atomoxetine (Strattera): Targets the brain chemical norepinephrine. It can develop attention and reduce impulsivity

	improving alertness and reducing hyperactivity and impulsivity	and hyperactivity. Alpha-2 adrenergic: How they operate in the brain to assist with ADHD is unclear. However, they minimize attention deficit disorder and impulsivity. They might likewise boost interest.
How rapidly They Start And Stop Working	Fast performing. A youngster will feel results within 30 to 90 minutes of the very first dosage, depending upon the medicine as well as individual sensitivity.	Atomoxetine (Strattera): Takes two to 4 weeks for the drug to have complete results. Kids can be reduced swiftly, generally within a few days. Alpha-2 adrenergic: Takes

		two weeks to understand if the medicine works. Children's overdoses over the long-term might require to be lessened gradually to avoid side effects when the drug is stopped.
	These drugs-- and their impacts-- leave the system within three to 12 hrs, relying on whether they're short-acting or long-acting.	
Dosing Frequency	Extended-release pills last six to 12 hours-- adequate to cover the school day	Atomoxetine (Strattera): Once, sometimes two times, a day Alpha-2 adrenergic: From one to 3 times a day.
Common Side Effects	Loss of appetite, difficulty sleeping	Atomoxetine (Strattera): Moodiness.

| | (Uncommon adverse effects consist of boosted stress and anxiety, agitation, frustrations, tics, psychosis.). | (Uncommon adverse effects include nausea or vomiting, anorexia nervosa, slowness.).

Alpha-2 adrenergic: Sleepiness, exhaustion.

(Uncommon adverse effects consist of loss of appetite, drop in high blood pressure, queasiness.) |
|---|---|---|
| Danger | Could cause weight management and possibly impact elevation. (Weight, as well | Atomoxetine (Strattera): Scarce incidence of liver difficulties. |

	as height, should be monitored.). Use with care in kids with pre-existing heart conditions since these medications can, in uncommon instances, create problems. A cardiologist ought to authorize the youngster taking it.	Alpha-2 adrenergic: May cause dizziness as well as passing out if it significantly impacts high blood pressure.
Efficiency	It improves interest as well as decreases impulsivity as well as attention deficit disorder	Atomoxetine (Strattera): Improves interest and also lowers impulsivity and attention deficit disorder in about 50 percent of

| | in 70 to 80 percent of patients. | patients.

Alpha-2 adrenergic: Reduces impulsivity as well as attention deficit disorder in 60 percent of patients. |
| Doctors Might recommend These Drugs | Generally, this is the first line of medical therapy for kids with ADHD and ADD. | Atomoxetine (Strattera): Maybe prescribed if a youngster can't endure the side effects of stimulants. It may also be an alternative for teens as well as young adults that may benefit from 24-hour coverage.

Alpha-2 adrenergic: Most |

		frequently utilized in addition to stimulants to help youngsters with severe signs.

HELPFUL TIPS FOR RAISING KIDS WITH ADHD

Obtain a little self-centered

Research studies reveal that parental stress may boost when increasing a kid with ADHD (mainly when various other conditions are likewise existing), which can result in many more parenting battles down the road.

Sometimes it takes a scientific study with substantial information to remind us stress, overload, and also exhaustion is real as well as not some imperfection we can will away.

In a globe where your youngster always comes first, you need to schedule in minutes that prioritize you.

Whatever that resembles-- a stroll with your canine, kickball with close friends, a foamy cappuccino, krav maga, or a face-first-in-the-pillow nap-- trust us when we say focusing on yourself will help you be a better parent.

2. Self-control your kid the same, but different

Children with ADHD need a somewhat various method, which suggests you require to be adaptable.

Your pal's child is tossing playthings and battling his teddy bear after recess. Typical parenting code would undoubtedly consider this time-out deserving. It's the very same for youngsters with ADHD, however not.

Since hyperactivity is a sign and symptom of ADHD, this behavior is often an outcome of their problem. It doesn't mean if they are feel untouchable- you require to select the proper penalty and also strategy.

Yelling at a youngster for their ADHD-related actions does not help them create the abilities they need to self-regulate, as well as they might wind up acting out much more if they feel they'll get chewed out regardless.

Attempt penalties, like a break, that feel routine, structured, and also give clear guidelines regarding why the habits aren't alright.

3. Produce as well as stick to a routine

Regimens are your youngster's buddy now.

You do not need to box them in with regulations on guidelines, but many kids with ADHD thrive under an established routine since they haven't found out how to prioritize points on their own.

It mainly applies to your routines before and after school.

While walking the stroll is most important, you can increase down on that organizing power by hanging a completely dry get rid of board schedule someplace famous in your house, like the kitchen.

Track your family members' to-do's, visits, and vital things to remember. If your child is mature enough for a tablet, phone, or computer system, try establishing digital pointers as well as signals.

Not only will your kid feel concentrated as well as support, yet it'll keep you responsible, also.

4. Establish clear guideline-- and also really follow them

Remember our speak about routines? It also applies to fundamental rules in your home.

It helps to reduce complications your child could have regarding actions, such as leaving the table throughout mealtimes. You can even ask your youngster to help set a few of these policies once they're old sufficient.

5. Take things one step at a time

Taking it to slow down can educate your youngster a more important lesson: mindfulness.

Sure it seems chic; however in addition to various other om-worthy advantages, science has located mindfulness to be efficient at minimizing ADHD signs and symptoms.

By selecting a straightforward job, like placing publications back on a shelf, and persevering from start to finish, you help your teen exercise their very own ability to concentrate.

Avoid giving them numerous tasks at a time, as well as do your finest to be a client.

6. Focus on play and also exercise

There's boosting proof that exercise can help kids with ADHD.

By advertising neural development as well as cognitive development, researches recommend that getting your children proceeding a regular basis might help minimize some of their signs and symptoms.

You'll establish them up for a healthy and balanced, active life.

7. Make dish prep ADHD-friendly

While there's no definitive study, numerous parents discover that sticking to particular dietary limitations can help alleviate some of their kid's ADHD signs.

A healthy and balanced diet regimen consisting of fresh vegetables and fruits, whole grains, as well as lean proteins is good for everybody.

However, parents might likewise take into consideration removing or reducing certain foods and components, consisting of yet not restricted to sugary foods and ones with artificial shades as well as chemicals.

You can also try adding more omega-3 fats-- also known as fish, nuts, and even seeds.

8. Perfect the art of the kickback

K, so you're not the God Father, yet incentivizing tasks will certainly produce a positive organization with cleansing, something several kids with ADHD deal with.

If you've ever before explained your kid's space as looking like a bomb went off, you understand what we indicate below.

To maintain that room tidy, you require to initial lead by instance.

Do your ideal to keep points at home clean, in spite of how appealing it is to let the recipes soak for another two days. Then, draw out the kickbacks incentives.

Ideally, these won't impact your kid's routines, so try points like allowing them to select the after-dinner movie or a factors system that adds up to a new toy, publication, or thing of clothes.

9. Make going to bed a special event

You don't need us to tell you that sleep essential for growing youngsters, yet it bears repeating: Sleep is so effing crucial for your youngster's growth and administration of their ADHD.

The trouble? Kids with ADHD are susceptible to rest concerns, especially if they are taking medication for their condition. To battle this, focus on healthy sleep patterns for your family.

That consists of having a set going to bed, possibly offering melatonin (ask your doc regarding how to do this properly), and switching off screens about a half hr before bed.

10. When unsure, try behavior therapy

Ask your pediatrician to attach you with a therapist who can educate you about behavior therapy.

Because moms and dads have such a substantial impact on their youngsters, it is most useful that children get their therapy directly from them.

A few sessions with an expert will reveal to you how to give positive interaction, positive support, framework, and also discipline for your child.

11. If you have an older youngster, do not hesitate to let someone else action in

Every parent loves the day their infant ends up being a teen, as well as World War III, erupts in their house.

Reality: This occurs to everybody, as well as you're * not * alone.

Reality 2: ADHD makes this turmoil even more challenging to browse, both for you and your kid.

Enter behavior modification 2.0. For children in middle school and also senior high school, a specialist could be the very best individual to help them navigate their signs and symptoms.

This kind of therapy delivered by a neutral third party can be specifically practical for children presenting defiance and also resistance (which is basically what teen roadways are led with).

Ask your doctor for a specialist recommendation. Not only can they help your teen, however, but they'll also have plenty of tips for maintaining an open discussion about treatment and ways to show judgment-free support.

12. Speak with your kid's teachers, but don't be a helicopter moms and dad

Teachers spend concerning seven hrs a day with your kids at school. Shouldn't you give them all the devices to make the most of those hours?

First things first, chat with your youngster's educators and care providers about your youngster's diagnosis. Probabilities are this isn't their very first rodeo, and also they'll recognize how to continue.

Enter prepared to answer inquiries as well as offer descriptions, yet do not turn the meeting into an hour-long ADHD 101 program.

The objective is to allow any individual caring for your youngster to leave with an understanding of how to stay up to date with well-established regimens, recognize triggers, and also make a plan to help your youngster flourish.

Maintain having these conversations frequently so that everyone stays on the same web page. Your kid's teacher could even have fresh ADHD parenting ideas from their very own communications with your kid.

13. For extra support in school, consider an IEP or Section 504

When the traditional educational program isn't sufficing, conversation with your child's school concerning producing an Independent Education Plan.

If they are not qualified for an IEP, you might still have the ability to obtain help using Section 504, which needs colleges to supply assistance to trainees with learning specials needs.

Keep in mind that you'll need a diagnosis from your kid's doctor in advance.

Additionally, be honest with your kid before making the change. No person wants to be selected as different in school, yet if your little one is battling, a tailored understanding plan can be simply what they need.

14. Let them fidget

Some kids focus far better when they have an electrical outlet for their fidgeting. You've become aware of fidget rewriters, but there's, in fact, a vast world of fantastic fidget-friendly playthings available.

Offering your youngster an outlet throughout moments when they're asked to sit still can help them concentrate much better in your home and at school (after you check with their teacher, obviously).

15. Demand designated seats

We understand we said not to be a helicopter mom and dad, but in this instance, going the extra mile can be valuable. An ADHD trainee's seat should be purposefully put within a classroom.

Deal with their teacher to locate an appropriate area, such as near the instructor, near the front of the classroom, or away from way too many distractions.

16. Take your kid to yoga exercise

Whether you take part with each other or authorize them up for a youngsters' yoga collection, make time to go on.

A regular yoga exercise practice has been revealed to lower symptoms of ADHD and has generally been confirmed efficient for dealing with issues like anxiousness and anxiety.

17. Try out vital oils

The science is still mediocre right here, as well as it's certainly not a substitute for legit therapies like behavior therapy. Yet, necessary oils are one more path numerous parents of children with ADHD speak highly of.

Oils like rosemary, peppermint, and lavender have actually all been connected to leisure and boosted concentration. Attempt establishing a diffuser while your youngster does homework or including a few drops to their bathroom water.

Just be cautious to avoid call with eyes, as well as do not apply to skin without diluting in the bathroom or a provider oil.

18. Make technology your close friend

As a parent, it's just natural to have made complicated feelings concerning display time. Still, if they're going to have electronic devices, you could as well utilize the sources available on them.

Younger kids will benefit from you taking the lead in assisting them to remain organized with their research, jobs, and also extracurriculars.

Yet older teenagers can take advantage of making use of these on their own to track tasks, part-time work schedules, university exams, study sessions, athletic contests, and also a lot more.

19. Look inside their head

Ever before, wish you could know what's taking place inside your youngster's head? Some individuals have discovered success in treating ADHD symptoms with neurofeedback.

This sort of training permits a youngster to actually see exactly how their brain responds to the job of focus, and also might help them discover far better tactics for remaining focused.

20. Spend even more time outside

Studies have revealed that time outdoors is beneficial for all, but a lot more so for youngsters with ADHD, who frequently have a much easier time concentrating after investing a little time in nature.

21. Display display time

Pun not meant. A lot more study is needed, however limiting screen time can help maintain ADHD signs and symptoms at bay.

Some researches recommend that kids and also teenagers with ADHD are more vulnerable to evaluate dependency problems, so it's finest to keep an eye out for extreme phone or computer system use.

Try going with a walk, playing a video game, or exercising a brand-new skill with all that additional free time.

22. Keep an open mind concerning medication

We do not criticize anyone for looking for ADHD treatments that do not involve drugs, but you require to be open to the possibility that they may be necessary eventually.

Talk with your youngster's doctor to try and also figure out the very best Rx for them, as well as do your research study, as well. If something does not appear right with one medication, it's your right as your kid's supporter to seek out second opinions.

Many children do thrive when the appropriate combination of medications is suggested, yet these need always to be taken as a component of a broader, customized therapy strategy.

On the whole, parents raising youngsters that have ADHD have a lot of options when it pertains to managing their kid's signs and symptoms.

Coming to be an educated as well as an included parent is the first step, followed by developing an active support group through therapists, doctors, teachers, and also other caregivers.

Make sure your young person always recognizes that you're on their side, which you'll do every little thing you can to support them as they browse life with ADHD.

And also, do not forget to remember to take care of yourself. Even taking a couple of minutes to high-five yourself will make you a far better parent day in day out.

The Myths and also Facts About ADHD.

Attention deficit disorder has been commonly questioned over for the last number of years as more and more kids are being diagnosed. Some individuals believe that people with ADHD slouch, stupid, and absence will power. Nonetheless, ADHD has been identified by the National Institute of Health and also the United States division of Education as a naturally based disorder. Most often, ADHD is identified in kids; however,r, since 1978, grownups have been formally diagnosed with grown-up ADHD too. It is obvious especially because the majority of children who are identified with ADHD will undoubtedly mature with the very same condition. To much better understand ADHD in its entirety, you require to comprehend what is a misconception as well as what is the reality.

MYTH-ADHD is not a genuine issue. ADHD is an absence of self-control.

FACT-ADHD is a neuro-behavioral developing problem. It is a chemical imbalance in the management systems of the brain. ADHD is a legit diagnosis by significant medical, emotional, and also educational organizations utilize the Diagnostic and Statistical Manual of Mental Disorders. It is likewise recognized by the NIH as well as the United States Department of

Education as a naturally based chemical discrepancy of natural chemicals in the brain.

MYTH- ADHD only influences boys.

FACT- Boys and girls are equally as most likely to be influenced by ADHD. There is nothing tried and tested that either sex is more likely to be impacted.

MYTH- Children with ADHD at some point outgrow their problem.

REALITY- Approximately 70% of children detected with ADHD will remain to have signs and symptoms up through teenage years as well as 60% will continue to experience symptoms right into their adult years.

MYTH- ADHD is an outcome of bad parenting.

REALITY- Parenting does not create ADHD. Children with ADHD can not manage the impulses that make them wayward. They are not instructed to act in this manner; it is the chemistry in the brain. Some parenting methods can improve the intensity of the symptoms.

MYTH- You can not have ADHD as an adult if you weren't identified as a child.

TRUTH- Some children are undiagnosed, or misdiagnosed throughout the childhood years. Others can manage their symptoms as a kid, consequently not ultimately experiencing or acknowledging their signs and symptoms till the adult years. The medical diagnosis of ADHD is prevalent and also ample.

MISCONCEPTION- It is impossible to detect ADHD in adults precisely.

FACT- Although there isn't one test that medical diagnosis ADHD in adults. The Diagnostic, Statistical Manual of Mental Disorders and American Medical Association papers, as well as the checklist's signs and symptoms of ADHD in both kids and also grownups and medical professionals, have particular standards on detecting such problems.

MYTH- People with ADHD are stupid as well as careless.

FACT- Many people with ADHD have above common knowledge. The inequalities in the brain cause symptoms, which make the individual look like they are stupid or careless. Many fabulous individuals are believed to have had ADHD. Individuals who can effectively manage their condition have gone on to be CEOs as well as owners of a business that are still successful today.

MYTH- Everyone experiences signs of ADHD eventually; smart individuals can conquer these signs and symptoms.

FACT- ADHD has nothing to do with intelligence. Many individuals with ADHD are exceptionally highly smart. Every person can experience symptoms of ADHD. In individuals without ADHD, it's typically due to overstimulation, attitude, mood, or exhaustion. For individuals that experience ADHD, they are continuously harmed by their symptoms.

MYTH-Someone with ADHD can not be depressed, nervous, or have psychological troubles.

TRUTH- Someone with ADHD is six times as most likely to experience an additional psychological or finding out condition.

MISCONCEPTION- ADHD medicine creates people to abuse medications.

FACT- The prescription medicine utilized for the therapy of ADHD has been verified secure and efficient. It is more likely that neglected people with ADHD have a higher threat to misuse medicines due to habit-forming propensities. Treatment lowers the risk.

CONCLUSION

In the past, ADHD (attention-deficit/hyperactivity condition) was thought about a problem that children had, and after that, "outgrew" before they maturated. However, we now understand that ADHD is a neurological condition that spans a lifetime.

The signs and symptoms of ADHD do change with time, nonetheless. Youth hyperactivity might decrease as an adult locates healthy and balanced methods to direct their power.

Even with the shift in symptoms, ADHD can still get in the way with an adult's performance. Relationships, health, work, and funds are just a couple of locations of a person's life that might be influenced.

ADHD usually goes undiagnosed for quite some time. Numerous grownups, who have felt "careless" or "scatter-brained," are surprised to find out that they have ADHD.

Whether you're a mom and dad who believes your kid has ADHD or you've just been identified with ADHD as a grown-up, it's essential to understand your symptoms, therapy choices, as well as the most effective techniques for living well with ADHD.

Do Not Go Yet; One Last Thing To Do

If you enjoyed this book or found it useful, I'd be very grateful if you'd post a short review on Amazon. Your support does make a difference, and I read all the reviews personally so I can get your feedback and make this book even better.

Thanks again for your support!

www.ingramcontent.com/pod-product-compliance
Lightning Source LLC
Chambersburg PA
CBHW070532220526
45467CB00003B/934